"This is a book filled with ...
it is about living with cancer ...
it too emotional and ev ...
Because it is about life ...
people don't do until th ...
think everyone should i ...
learn from Lisa's wisdom and experience rather than their own difficulties.

"It is a beautiful love story of soul mates and natives who learn what it is like to live with pain while loving life. I wish everyone could live their experience frightening as it may be to many. If you have the courage to read on you will laugh, cry and experience all the things that life holds in store for us. It is like group therapy with true survivors. Survival and beating cancer are not about being cured of the disease. They are about qualities that people reveal in the face of adversity. Learn them from Lisa's story.

"We all die though we hate to admit it. Don't wait for the reality to set in before you wake up to the true joys of life. Read on and start to live now. It's a shame to waste your lifetime."

—**Bernie Siegel, M.D.**
author of *Love, Medicine and Miracles*
and *Prescriptions for Living*

"A moving account of a personal journey through sadness, fear, courage and triumph shared by a cancer patient who was very unfortunate to be diagnosed with this disease when she was too young, but became fortunate enough to win the battle and tell her story."

—**Anas Younes, M.D.**
oncologist at the world-renowned MD Anderson
Cancer Center

"*Only When I Sleep* is Lisa Brawley's triumphant account of her journey through Hodgkin's lymphoma. Honest and insightful, Lisa describes the practical, emotional, social and spiritual challenges of being a twenty-four-year-old, newly married woman with cancer. This is as much a story of family love as of personal growth through adversity."

—Wendy Harpham, M.D., F.A.C.P.
author of *Diagnosis: Cancer, After Cancer*
and *When a Parent Has Cancer*

ONLY WHEN I SLEEP

My Family's Journey Through Cancer

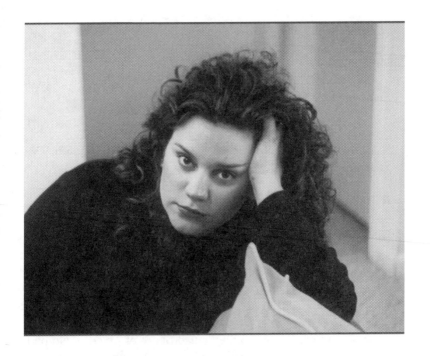

Lisa Shaw-Brawley

Foreword by Robert Urich

Health Communications, Inc.
Deerfield Beach, Florida

www.hci-online.com

Library of Congress Cataloging-in-Publication Data

Shaw-Brawley, Lisa, date.
    Only when I sleep : my family's journey through cancer / Lisa
Shaw-Brawley, with a foreword by Robert Urich.
        p. cm.
    ISBN 1-55874-774-5 (trade paper)
        1. Shaw-Brawley, Lisa, date—Health. 2. Lymphomas—
Patients—United States—Biography. I. Title

RC280.L9 S52 2000
362.1'9699446'0092—dc 21
[B]

                                                                00-021152

©2000 Lisa Shaw-Brawley
ISBN 1-55874-774-5

Publisher: Health Communications, Inc.
                3201 S.W. 15th Street
                Deerfield Beach, FL 33442-8190

Cover design by Larissa Hise
Inside book design by Dawn Grove
Cover color photos of author by Wes Brawley
Cover black-and-white photo of author by Marilyn Brodwick

To my parents.

I am so fortunate to have the people
who brought me into the world
also help take care of me in the world.

And to Wesley.

I have known you most of my life,
and I have loved you all of that time.

Your love sustains me.

Acknowledgments

This book was published because of the people who believed in its message and in me as the storyteller.

I am thankful to my lifelong family physician, Dr. William McCabe, for his no-nonsense approach to caring for my family over the years and for sending me to Dr. Verma, my treating oncologist, when the X-ray pointed to cancer. I thank Dr. Ajay Verma for bringing clarity to my diagnosis and to what was necessary of me to fully recover. And I thank Mary Trevor, my oncology nurse throughout treatment, for always knowing just what I needed exactly when I needed it. She made Tuesdays more bearable. I thank Dr. Vidya Bobba, my radiology oncologist, for getting me through the final stretch of my treatment safely and with care. I also thank Dr. Anas Younes, my follow-up oncologist, for continuing to look after me. With each check-up I get stronger and need less of his time, but I always know he will make time for me when I do need it.

Mere words could not convey the gratitude I feel toward my agent Carole Bidnick. She believed that my story was worth telling, and I will always be grateful for her faith in me. Carole was the essential beginning of what I know was the ultimate journey as an author, and I am honored to call her my friend.

In survivorship, I thank Robert Urich for his contribution of the foreword. Enlisting his help taught me a lesson in perseverance. Today and twenty years from now, when this book rests on my bookshelf at home, I will always cherish his words of endorsement.

I also thank John Wall, Mr. Urich's manager and friend, for being available to me during the long process of this book's creation.

I thank my editorial team at Health Communications. I thank Matthew Diener for believing in the purpose of this book and for putting such a marvelous support system in place for the editing process. And I thank Lisa Drucker for answering all of my questions and for the kind words that put me at ease from the start. I feel blessed to have been placed with a publishing house of such integrity.

I am grateful to my copy editor, Erica Orloff, for choosing to work on my book from the list of others. Once again, I was sent the perfect match for the work that lay ahead.

I thank writing consultant Dorothy Wall for her expertise and for helping me put together the proposal that made them all want to read more.

I thank Susan Page, not only for writing *The Shortest Distance Between You and a Published Book,* which I read numerous times, but also for taking my calls after I read it and for referring me to Carole and Dorothy. She couldn't have realized at the time what a gift she was giving me.

I thank Juliette Wittman for helping me find creative ways to remain in school while writing the manuscript.

I also thank Dr. Bernie Siegel, Dr. Wendy Harpham and Dr. Anas Younes for supporting this book early on. I am honored by their approval and support of my work.

I thank Mrs. Petersen, my senior-year English teacher, for the time she told me that reading my journal entries was much like reading a novel. Teachers are supposed to help shape young lives, and she was the first person I believed when being told I was a talented writer.

I give many thanks to my family and friends who read and re-read the early drafts and helped me get it right before sending it out into the literary world.

On behalf of my family, I would like to thank every positive person we encountered during the most arduous time in our lives. We thank them for contributing to the triumph during the tragedy.

I thank Wesley's family: Donna and Roger Burton, for their support and for believing in us enough to give the gift of their contribution to this book's potential success; and Jimbo Carroll for his generosity which enabled us to move through my treatment with few outside worries.

I thank my dad for the words he contributed to this book. I hope the sensitivity in his writing will help many parents realize they are not alone. I wonder if this is what he had in mind when he wrote, "Go get 'em, honey!" in my got-well party guest book?

I am thankful for my wonderful mother and can only pray that I will grow to have her gift of selflessness. May I become the mother that she has always been to me.

Most of all, I thank my husband Wesley. I thank him for continuing to be my focal source of strength long after he chose to leave cancer behind. I could not and would not have done this without him.

Foreword

I first met Lisa back in September of 1997 when I was the keynote speaker at a patient conference held annually by MD Anderson Cancer Center. During a press conference held shortly before I was scheduled to speak, she approached me in a room full of reporters. Lisa told me that she'd had Hodgkin's disease and that she was one of the thousands of people who had sent a letter to me when hearing I had been diagnosed with synovial sarcoma. It was during our first meeting that Lisa told me she was writing a book about her own cancer experience. She gave a few chapters to my manager John Wall and asked that I review them and consider writing the foreword for her book. Included with the chapters was a letter from her husband, an excerpt from the chapter her father had written, and photographs of her and her family taken at her got-well party. I was touched by what I read, so I sent a note to her asking that she send me her book when it was ready.

Many people talk about writing books only to find what an enormous challenge it is. And for that reason, I didn't really give much thought to Lisa's book over the next year. It wasn't until I saw her again a year later at another patient conference and she told me that her book was being published that I discovered her life's ambition to be an author would actually be realized.

After having endured my own battle against cancer, I considered the strength she must have had to face it at such a young age. She was only twenty-four years old, almost half my age, when she was diagnosed. But, like I had, she had the most critical components in place when fighting cancer: family support, a competent medical team and the gift of hope. And now, she has found the strength to write it all down, trying to reach others with the story of her family's journey through cancer.

I have traveled all over the country talking to people who have also endured cancer, and talking about it unleashes an army of support. I tell my own story of survival and draw strength from theirs. The survivorship I share with them is truly more abundant than any other form of celebrity I have known. I received such an enormous outpouring of support from thousands of people internationally, and it wasn't long before I realized that the love and support I received was in large measure what moved me toward recovering. It is Lisa's prayer that, with her story of survival, she will be able to help those who are just beginning their own battle. There is nothing like the voice of a survivor when fear of the unknown comes taunting.

When being diagnosed with cancer, the most that one can really begin to hope for is another day to come and the strength to wake up and participate fully in that day. There are no guarantees, but, if you're fortunate, you move beyond the fear and learn to live with what has come to your life. You learn to search for things inside yourself, finding what is authentic and true for your own life. Your family becomes even more important than before, and your gift of life and survival slowly becomes real again. Lisa has experienced one of the best possible outcomes. She not only beat the cancer, but she also went on to accomplish some of the most important goals in her life. Lisa has learned to not waste time but to move forward with the gift she was given.

So many times, after overcoming obstacles large and small in our lives, we tend to forget about the promises we made to ourselves and to others while in the midst of it, but I have tried never to do that. Because of this, I am reminded of a quote from psychiatrist Carl Jung: "Conflict engenders fire. The fire of passions and effects. And like all fire, it has two properties. That of combustion and that of creating light." And I thought that if I could somehow survive the combustion aspect of this medical event in my life, then maybe it could be the source of spiritual illumination. And that's why I wanted to write this for Lisa, because we are all on a healing journey. The family Lisa has today would be enough, but in her attempts to help others better cope with what is likely to be the most difficult time in their lives, she has given the gift of her own story. We can all strive to gain as much hard-earned wisdom in our own journeys. We can all hope to bask in the love of our families; to prove science wrong by creating other miracles in our lives; and to take time to share the hope with others. This book is Lisa's gift of hope to all of us.

In Survivorship,
Robert Urich

One

Christmas Night, 1995

I should be in bed. It's after midnight, so Christmas is officially over. As much as I have come to accept living further away from my family, it always feels good to be home.

I write by the only light in the room: a glowing angel atop the Christmas tree and the colored, blinking lights draped from limb to limb. We trimmed it just two days ago. Traditionally, we would cut down our own tree Thanksgiving weekend on my Grandma and Grandpa Shaw's mountaintop property, but with my Grandpa, so many cherished traditions have died.

My dad describes this year's tree as the Charlie Brown Christmas tree. The few branches it does possess are frail and have few pine needles. It has already begun to dry out. My parents have never been very particular about the tree that we trim, because they have always said it's the people who live here who light up our home. When my brother and I used to anxiously ask how we should begin decorating each

1

year, my mother would say, "Decorate the tree the way you've decorated our lives."

There were times in my life that my brother and I would each receive only one gift from my parents, because that was all they could afford. The gift was always something we desperately wanted, like alloy rims for my brother's slowly built BMX bike or the typewriter I begged for that weighed more than I did and was just as loud. No matter the gift, we learned early on the meaning of Christmas. Even as the years passed and my father began to earn substantially more money, we never made Christmas lists or expected Santa to bring us everything we asked for throughout the year. We loved the gifts, but I think even at that young age, we just felt lucky to have each other.

One of my best friends used to come to our house Christmas morning and show me all of her gifts, but I never got jealous. This is the same friend whose mother was on her third marriage to a man that she didn't love but who did provide the gifts that appeared under their tree each year. I knew my life was richer. She probably did, too, because she usually spent the rest of the day at our house with my family rather than her own.

Since Wesley and I moved to Texas in early 1994, we have promised to return every other year for the holidays. There's something very special about waking up in the only home I remember living in as a child and being able to have Wesley and our dog, Huck, here with me. When I was a child, we lived in the smaller house two doors down before my parents had this one built. The times I spend awake while everyone else sleeps are always spent reflecting on the years I lived here.

I just finished watching a television interview with Naomi Judd. She was talking about remaining in remission from hepatitis C, attributing it to her spirituality, taking care of herself physically and having a positive attitude. I honestly don't know how she does it. To have something so wrong with you it could take your life—I can't imagine. I've always heard the saying about God not giving people more than they can handle, but I don't believe that always holds true. I have suffered little in my life, which makes me more vulnerable to life's unpredictable possibilities. Only in the face of genuine tragedy do most people learn of the human spirit's promise. I don't think I could be so strong.

As much as I enjoy spending time alone while everyone else sleeps, I am mainly still awake because I can't stop itching. I thought for sure it was the laundry detergent or the water at home, but after washing my clothes and showering at Wesley's mom's house last week, I don't know what it could be.

I guess I will go to bed. I think I will go see Dr. McCabe tomorrow since I am here. Early tonight, I discovered that my glands are still swollen from a few weeks ago, and I just noticed another gland swollen between my collarbone and my neck. The lump is small, smaller than a golf ball, but it wasn't there earlier today. He'll be able to give me some antibiotics to lessen the swelling.

I woke Wesley up to feel the lump and asked him if I should go to the doctor. He said I should if it'll make me feel better. I'll try getting in to see Dr. McCabe tomorrow, while Wesley and my dad are golfing. It's better than waiting until we go back to Texas. I feel more comfortable with my doctor. After all, he did deliver me twenty-four years ago.

Two

December 26, the next day . . .

8:52 P.M.—As I lie here in bed, I keep asking myself if any of this is real. How stupid and naive I was to think Dr. McCabe would give me antibiotics and send me home.

I sat in Dr. McCabe's office and waited over an hour to see him. I didn't mind. I expected to wait. I hadn't been to see him since he diagnosed me with gallstones two years ago. Wesley and I had only been married for twelve days when I had my gallbladder removed. It wasn't exactly our idea of a honeymoon, but I felt much better after the surgery. That is one of the reasons I didn't mind waiting for my doctor. Every time I have gone to see him, he knows what is wrong with me, and then he fixes it. I've heard other people complain about their family doctor not treating them properly for what ails them, but I have never experienced that with him.

The wait was boring, so I sat and "people watched." Most of the patients were at least sixty years old and sat in their chairs reading magazines, trying not to fall asleep. It's been years since Dr. McCabe stopped delivering babies. My

5

brother, Vance, was one of the first babies he delivered. My mom had a different doctor at the beginning of her pregnancy, but that doctor died when she was seven months pregnant with my brother. Dr. McCabe has been our family doctor ever since. Some of my relatives go to him as well. My Grandma Shaw used to, until she got tired of waiting. She wrote him a nasty letter about how inconsiderate it was of him to make his patients sometimes wait in the lobby for several hours. She not-so-politely informed him that she'd be taking her business elsewhere. Until my grandpa's death, he continued seeing Dr. McCabe, despite my grandma's feelings. My grandpa made the right choice. When my grandpa was bed-ridden in the last days of his life, Dr. McCabe called our family at my grandparents' home to see how he was doing. He wanted to make sure my grandpa's pain was being well-managed. Beyond the familiarity I had always known with Dr. McCabe, I knew then that a doctor who made house calls was worth waiting for.

I sat in the office and wondered what each person was there for. A woman walked into the lobby and rushed outside crying. A man followed her, and the two of them sat in their car smoking a cigarette. I hoped they weren't told one of them had lung cancer. You never know; after all, my grandpa never smoked a day in his life and he died of lung cancer. He was a diesel mechanic most of his life and was also exposed to asbestos, but if you asked him, my grandpa would have told you he would not have changed how he earned his living. He provided for his family.

My appointment was for 11:00 A.M., but I didn't have my vitals checked until after noon. I overheard the gentleman who ran outside talking to a nurse. He was being admitted to the hospital for a minor injury. He'd fallen down in a drunken stupor. I felt sorry for his wife.

That was what had the doctor running behind, admitting

two patients to the hospital. I still didn't mind waiting. I was lucky to have gotten in so quickly. When I woke up this morning, Wesley had already told my dad about the lump. My dad misunderstood him, thinking the lump was in my breast. Poor guy. I bet that scared him until Wesley clarified that the lump was in my neck and was probably just swollen glands. The next thing I knew, my dad was telling me he got me an appointment with Dr. McCabe.

I was glad to find out I had lost a few pounds. Lately, with very little effort, I have managed to shed some of the weight I have been trying to lose for months.

I finally managed to see Dr. McCabe around 1:00 P.M. He walked in and started with his usual small talk, asking how my family was doing. I reciprocated. Then, he asked what brought me in to see him.

"I've had swollen glands for a few weeks, and last night I noticed another gland has swelled. It's between my neck and my collar bone," I explained.

He stood in front of me and started feeling the glands in my neck. He saw the lump and felt his way to it.

While he stood before me, I studied the lines that had accumulated on his face and the hair that had changed from black to gray in my lifetime. He was still handsome, still ran four days a week, and still tirelessly contested the statistic claiming that many doctors die of a heart attack from stress before they are old enough to retire. It looked like he was still winning.

"That's a lymph node. It shouldn't be swollen at any time for any reason," he said as he backed away. He pulled his swiveling stool over to me and sat down. With his hands folded tightly around his kneecap, he bent his left knee and leaned back. "Have you been having any night sweats or losing unexplained weight lately?"

"No, what are night sweats?" I asked, still unconcerned.

"You'd know if you were having them. So you haven't lost any weight lately?" he asked again.

"Not unexplained. Why? What would cause my lymph node to swell?" I knew I had lost some weight but my appetite had decreased lately; I assumed it was just because of my hectic schedule. Surely this weight loss had nothing to do with the lump. I didn't want to tell him about it. I was starting to get frightened.

"Well, it could be a few things, but it may be Hodgkin's disease."

"What's Hodgkin's disease?" I asked. I'd heard about a hockey player who'd had it. But then I thought it might be some type of blood disease.

"It's a disease that's very easily treated if found early, especially if it's above the diaphragm. We'll draw some blood here today and also do a chest X-ray. Then, I'll arrange for you to have an upper body CAT scan tomorrow."

"Blood drawn? Is that to check my white blood cell count?" I asked, remembering that test from the movies.

"Exactly, and it'll give us an idea about some other things as well," Dr. McCabe answered.

I got scared. In the movies, a white blood cell check meant you had cancer, but he hadn't mentioned the word cancer.

"What'll happen if I have it? Where would I get treated?" I asked. I felt the panic coming over me. It had to be a mistake.

"Let's just see what we find," Dr. McCabe said.

My first thought was that I would be going to the nearest pharmacy to pick up some medicine, but in case I was wrong, and it could get worse, I wanted to call Wesley. "I want my dad to bring my husband. I want him here with me."

"You can use this phone."

I dialed the phone while he sat in his swivel chair and jotted down his notes. I appreciated him staying with me while I called.

"Dad, would you bring Wesley up here?" I asked as soon as he answered.

"Sure, why?" he asked.

"Because Dr. McCabe is running some tests, and I want Wesley here with me. Would you bring him up now?"

"What does he think is wrong?"

"Now let's not get all worked up. Let's just wait and see what we find," Dr. McCabe interjected.

"Did you hear him, Dad?"

"What did he say?" my dad asked.

"He said for us not to worry, but will you please bring Wesley up here?" I requested again.

"Yeah, we're on our way."

"Leave now, okay?" I continued.

"Okay, we'll be right there."

"You'll tell Wesley what's going on?"

"Yeah," he reassured me.

"Okay. Hurry Dad."

"Okay. I love you, babe," he said.

"I love you," I told him before I hung up the phone.

"He's bringing him up here. What do I do?" I was so scared I could hardly stand.

"I'll take an X-ray of your chest, then while the pictures develop, the nurse will draw some blood."

"So you'll have a pretty good idea from the X-ray before I leave?" I couldn't bear waiting until later to find out something, anything.

"Yes, but we won't have the results of your blood work until this afternoon or maybe even tomorrow. Follow me."

And I did. I followed that man wherever he wanted me to go. I only saw him occasionally throughout the years, but he was the first person to ever hold me in his hands, so I put my life into them once again. I followed him to the X-ray room.

I didn't have to change my clothes, only take off my bra. I

was glad to do that. The bra made my itching worse.

"Okay, now stand against this metal slab and stand up real straight. Stand still until I tell you to relax."

I did as he said. When that picture was finished, he asked me to turn and face to my left, bend my elbows, and lift my arms out in front of me. It was in that motion I realized something was wrong inside of me. Something was really wrong. My chest felt tight inside, and when I held my arms up it suffocated my lungs. It was like there was no room for my lungs to hold my breath while he did the X-ray. I knew. And from that moment on, during each test they took, I knew it was not a matter of whether or not they'd find anything, but how much they would find. I put my head down and sighed out loud. I wanted to cry, but I didn't. It's not as if I am the type of person who is uncomfortable with crying, but it seemed too soon to cry. I felt too frightened to cry. I just followed Dr. McCabe to the next room, where the nurse was waiting to draw my blood.

"You have tiny veins, Lisa. They are hiding from me today. I'm going to try and raise them up," the nurse said as she spread something warm and gooey on the inside of my arm, where the largest vein was hiding.

As we sat there waiting for my veins to cooperate, I wondered if she knew something that I didn't. . . . If she felt sorry for me, because I was having those tests.

"It wouldn't be so bad to have my blood drawn if I were finding out I was pregnant or something," I confessed.

"I know, but we'll get you taken care of," she said. "Okay, a little prick now."

As she inserted the needle, I didn't watch. It hurt a little bit, but I didn't care. I just hoped Wesley would be there soon. The nurse had me wait in the back hall while the X-rays were developing. "Doctor will be back here in a minute. You can have a seat."

"My dad is bringing my husband up here. Will you send him back as soon as he arrives?" I didn't want to sit back there alone. Just then, another nurse came around the corner and Wesley was walking behind her.

"Here she is. Look who's here," the nurse said with a reassuring smile.

"Thank you," Wesley said as he sat down.

"Are you okay? What's going on?" Wesley asked.

"I don't know. Dr. McCabe did some X-rays and the nurse drew some blood," I explained.

"What do we do now?"

"I guess we wait for the X-rays to be done. She said the doctor will be with me in a minute."

As I sat there, I felt my heart beating faster than it ever had before. I tried to keep my feet steady on the floor, but I could not control them. They shook uncontrollably, until finally, my whole body was shaking. I began to feel cold, and my teeth were chattering.

"Try to calm down," Wesley said, as he put his hand on my thigh.

"I can't. Wesley, I know something is wrong. Something is really wrong." I barely got the words out through the chattering.

"You need to calm down. Nothing is wrong," he tried to reassure me as he picked up a magazine. I didn't take that as an inconsiderate move; I know my husband well. He's never been a worrier and rarely expects the worst.

"But I could feel it when I lifted my arms," I continued.

"Feel what?"

"Feel whatever it is inside of me," I answered, though I couldn't say the word.

"He'll be out in a minute. Just calm down until he tells us what is going on."

"Okay . . . okay," I reluctantly agreed.

"Here. Read a magazine," he said as he passed one my way, but I had no interest.

Wesley skimmed through his magazine. He didn't hear Dr. McCabe talking to the nurse around the corner, but I did.

"Here's her X-ray, Doctor," she said as she flipped on the light switch to show it to him.

And that was the moment everything changed for me. The moment my life became something different than it had ever been, filling me with an agony I had never known. In that moment, as he let out a loud whistle, expressing his amazement at what he saw on my chest X-ray, something inside of my spirit that I didn't even realize I had possessed was lost forever.

"Wesley, I have cancer!" I shook even more as the words somehow escaped my mouth. It was as if I had said them so slowly that I could have run a mile, sat back down next to myself, and still heard the words as they were spoken.

"What?"

"Didn't you hear him? It's bad. It's really bad!"

"What's bad?"

"He just saw my X-ray."

Wesley seemed confused. Just then, Dr. McCabe came around the corner and as he walked toward us, his words and his steps etched a difference in my life I cannot possibly explain.

"Lisa, I'm sure you have either Hodgkin's or non-Hodgkin's lymphoma. I'm ordering a full-body CAT scan for tomorrow and a biopsy on Thursday." To some, his directness may have seemed harsh, but to me, he was being my doctor.

"Is my X-ray bad?" I dared to ask.

"It's full of something, kid. Now we just have to find out what and where it is."

"What do I do now?" I asked, looking at Wesley and

realizing he was still very confused. Wesley's hazel eyes always turn greener when he cries or when he is extremely tired. Now I discovered the flecks of green also deepen in panic.

"They're on the phone now setting up an appointment for your CAT scan tomorrow, and we'll call you later with an appointment for the biopsy. If it's Hodgkin's, you've got a good chance of beating it. Let's just wait and see." Wesley hadn't spoken a word until Dr. McCabe offered his hand to shake it.

"Thank you, doctor. Do I just take her home now?"

"Yeah. Try not to worry. We'll get it figured out."

The two released hands, then we walked toward the front desk, where the receptionist was writing down information about the next day's CAT scan. Linda, one of the nurses, asked me if I'd been sick with a cold at all. I told her I hadn't. When she asked how long the lump had been there, I knew why she was asking. She probably figured from the looks of my X-ray that it had been there for a while, but I hadn't done anything about it.

I wanted to tell her, "You're crazy to think I'd go around with a lump like this on my neck and ignore it. I just felt it at 1:00 A.M. this morning, and here I am. I didn't wait. The cancer waited. It waited to show itself, and now maybe it's too late. Now maybe it's everywhere else. I came as soon as I could. And what good has that done me? It's all over the X-ray." But, I just said, "I haven't been sick at all," as I lowered my head. Wesley took the appointment card, and we both walked toward the door.

As we exited, I thought about the people sitting in the lobby, who were there to be treated for a common cold or minor injury. Earlier, I had wondered if any of them, being so old, were there to see the doctor about cancer or something else serious. I wondered if any of them were dying. As I left the building, I thought to myself, *No, Lisa. It's you who will leave here today with cancer. It's you who might be dying.* I went there this morning with what I thought were my swollen glands, but I left with cancer. When Wesley shut the door behind me, I knew my life was about to change.

Three

Still December 26 . . .

Wesley opened the car door for me, and as I was about to get inside, I took one last look at the building where Dr. McCabe's office has been all of my life. I thought about all of the years I had walked into his office with a cold or a feverish flu. I used to love reading the *Highlights* magazines that were on the table for children to keep themselves occupied. I always opened the magazine to the page where I could search for the items hidden within the picture. As we drove away, it saddened me to think of how innocently I had entered his office today, not knowing what was coming. I walked in there just as I had each time in the two-and-a-half decades before.

On the way home, Wesley and I didn't discuss what either of us was feeling about what had just taken place. We only spoke of the appointments that were set up for tomorrow. Always trying to shield me from negative thoughts, he tried to be optimistic and said he thought it would probably turn out to be nothing, but I think he knew that we were not going to be so lucky. We weren't going to get out of this without going through the struggle ahead of us. I knew what was coming. There was no denying it.

Soon, we were in my parents' driveway. I got out of the car and walked toward their front door. As I put my hand on the doorknob, I looked up at the engraved nameplate on the door that read, "Shaw's." It was then that I realized what I was about to do.

I hadn't even given any thought to how I would tell my parents the news. I knew it was important to be careful how I told them. This made me think about my grandpa and the one comfort that had helped my dad better cope with his father's departure. He said it on several occasions: "My father lived a full life, and most importantly, he never had to bury a child or a grandchild." We all took great comfort in that.

I knew my parents were incapable of losing one of their two children. Not that any parent is equipped to cope with such a loss, but I just kept hearing my dad say the words of my grandfather's good fortune. This was a day that would be deeply imbedded in their memory for the rest of their lives, and how I told them would make a difference. I took a deep breath and walked inside with my thoughts collected, as ready as I would ever be.

"I need to talk with both of you," I said to my dad. He was sitting on the far edge of the couch, watching football on television.

"Your mom is in the garage. What's up?" he asked.

"Just a minute, I have to get Mom," I replied. As I walked toward the garage door, I noticed a sticker of the Jetsons' family dog. It was in the left hand, bottom corner of the door. I hadn't noticed that sticker of the blue dog in years. I thought about all of the visitors through the years who had probably noticed it. But to us, it was just a part of the door, a part of the house, a reminder of something we put there as children. My mom refinished our bedroom doors long ago, after years of stickers being put on them in layers. I wondered if she had left this one sticker on the garage door on purpose, to remind us of the children we once were.

"Mom, I need to talk to you," I told her.

"What's wrong?" she asked as she transferred clothes from the washer to the dryer. When I saw her standing there, doing what I had found her doing so many times in my life, I wished to God I was opening that door to ask her if I could go down the street to play or tell her she had a phone call; anything other than what I had to do. Anything to spare this woman, my mother, who had washed my clothes all of my life and tucked me into bed every night, the pain she was about to feel.

"Please just come inside."

I backed away from the door and let it close on its own, as it always has. I walked toward the couch. My dad turned off the television. I found a place on the couch, and we waited for my mom to come inside. Wesley sat across from my dad and me. My mom entered the room and took a seat on the arm of the couch, sitting to the right of me. With my parents at my side and my husband close by, the words somehow managed to come out.

"I am scheduled for some tests tomorrow," I began. "Dr. McCabe thinks I have Hodgkin's disease."

"What's Hodgkin's disease?" my dad asked.

"Well, it's . . . it's cancer," I answered.

"What? What do you mean?" my mom asked as I heard the panic in her voice.

"What are the tests for?" my dad asked, equally panicked. My dad never worries unnecessarily, but I knew this time fear overcame him.

"I . . . I don't know." It was all too overwhelming.

My mother immediately began reaching, trying to find

something that could make this all be a mistake. "Well, did you tell them you've been itching? Did you tell them you haven't been eating much? Maybe it's something else. Maybe they're wrong."

"I don't know, Mom. I don't know," I answered. It was then that I cried for the first time since I had been told. My parents each put one of their arms around me and with their free hand, they held each other's.

I looked over at Wesley and saw him staring at the floor. I knew he was listening to every word we were saying, but to face us was too difficult for him. The moment became too much for me to bear. "I can't do this. I *cannot* do this," I said, more overwhelmed than I could manage.

"*We'll* do this. We'll do it together. We'll listen to Dr. McCabe. We trust him. He'll help us. He'll take care of you," my dad interjected, thinking I meant something other than I did. "You can do it. We'll fight it. We'll beat it."

I hadn't given any thought to what I would have to do in order to fight this disease. I just knew I couldn't sit there any longer and watch the pain my parents were in. I couldn't even feel my own pain. It was like I was standing outside of myself, watching all of it take place. Once again, I looked at Wesley and I could see his pain. I felt sad for what he was going through. Wesley had had other excruciating moments like this in his young life. It wasn't long ago that he, as the oldest of his siblings, was the one to ask his father if he wanted to be on life support if necessary. That was something no child should ever have to do, and he's never gotten over it. And now, here he sits listening to me tell my parents of cancer. When Wesley looked up at me, I could see the tears welling up in his eyes. He was overwhelmed, so he got up from the chair and walked out the same door my mom had entered just moments before.

In that instant, something inside of me switched; something

inside of me stopped hurting and started fighting. "Let's just wait and see what happens. Let's not worry about this. When Grandpa was waiting on tests, we all worried. When we did finally find out what was wrong with him, I wished I had enjoyed the time of not knowing. Let's just wait and see," I said to both of them.

I do have other reasons for wanting to wait. I am beginning to feel a cloud come over me, a layer of protection, possibly—something I believe is a blanket of fog from God to protect me from the uncertainties of cancer and allow me to question whether or not any of it is really happening.

I can also feel something else coming over me, something dark and reckless, and something that, once it arrives, will take my life in a direction I find inconceivable. And maybe it will lead me to a place that I can never escape from and will be my place of no return. Maybe it will be where I take my last breath in this world and then find myself only a memory to those I have loved and those who have loved me. Whatever it is, it is coming toward me at full speed, and I am fully aware of its presence. I am not in denial. I just need a couple more days to try and prepare. Just a couple more days before it becomes absolute.

My dad followed my lead and agreed, "Okay. We'll wait until the tests are done. We'll wait." My mom was still sitting next to me. I knew they were both holding in what would inevitably have to surface, the tears and the fear of what might happen to me. But I also knew they weren't going to let me see their fears.

The three of us sat quietly hugging. After a few moments, we released our embrace. Then I asked my dad to check on Wesley. I got up when he did, but before he left the room, I had one last thing to say, "Somebody needs to call Vance." My brother lived in Montana and needed to know before anyone else was told.

"I'll do it," my dad volunteered as he walked outside to find Wesley.

The two of them weren't outside very long. When they returned, they both seemed better.

"Are you okay?" I asked Wesley, feeling badly for him, knowing how scared he must be. The fear I saw in his face was so recognizable. It's the same pain I saw when his dad, Alton, died only one year ago. I thought about Alton, realizing how angry he would have been if he were still here and learned I might have cancer. And just as quickly, I remembered he was in heaven, allowing him to see what we see, but with the perfection of God's will. That made me smile. He knew more than we did, and I liked to think he already knew I would survive.

"I'm okay. You're going to be all right. Everything is going to be okay," he answered with conviction.

"It has to be," I responded.

My dad took the phone outside to call Vance and later came back inside with very swollen, red eyes. He said Vance would call me a little later. I wondered why he was waiting to talk with me, and then I realized he probably had to collect himself first. I told my parents and Wesley that I didn't want everyone to know about this until we knew what we were dealing with. We agreed there were some people we wanted to tell, but very few.

I called my friend, Sara, a little while ago. I also tried to call Bev, my foster sister, but she wasn't home. I told her husband Stan what was going on. I am leaving it up to my parents to call my grandmas. I don't mind if other members of the family are told, but I just don't have the energy to call everyone at this point.

9:46 P.M.—People started calling already. Both of my grandmas called earlier, wanting me to know they love me and telling me I'll be okay. Vance called soon after he and my dad spoke. He and Heather, his bride of two months, had company and wanted to wait until they left before calling me back. The conversations have gone very well with everyone. I was most surprised with Bev's reaction. I just talked with her, and she was much calmer than I thought she would be. Her closeness to God must really be changing her, because she isn't the same Bev I shared a bedroom with when I was five years old and she was thirteen. I am glad to know God is healing the hurts in her life.

I remember the day my parents discussed the possibility of taking Bev in as their foster child. Bev had been our baby-sitter for a few months. She lived two blocks away from our house with her four sisters and two brothers. The oldest child was only sixteen and the youngest was still in diapers. Her mother had left her children alone, so Child Protective Services found out and placed each of them in foster care. Bev was a good kid, considering the circumstances in which she grew up, and my parents wanted to help her if they could. I was thrilled with the idea. My parents told us not to mention it to her, because there were some things that had to be worked out before they could be sure they would be able to take her in. Bev baby-sat us later that night, and I remember she had a purple flower on her ear when she arrived. She picked me up, and the first words I blurted out to her were, "You're going to come and live with us!" My parents didn't seem surprised I hadn't kept our secret.

Bev wanted to live with us; so after the social worker inspected our home and interviewed each of us it became official. I had a sister, and even though she only lived with us less than a year, she has remained in our lives, and we continue referring to each other as sisters to this day.

Bev will be at my CAT scan tomorrow, even though I told her I wouldn't know anything yet. She said she wanted to be there to help in any way she could. I know Bev will be helpful to me. To tell the truth, I don't think I have a choice in the matter. She insisted on being there.

Tomorrow will begin the testing process, letting us know exactly what is going on inside of me. I am going to take a bath now. It's the only thing that gives me any relief from the constant itching I can't get rid of. I just hope I can sleep tonight.

Wednesday, December 27

When I woke up this morning, Wesley and I were holding hands. We must have fallen asleep that way. The last words I heard before I went to sleep last night were of Wesley telling me I would be okay and he loves me. Later, I found my mom reading a book about health and remedies for common ailments. I could tell she had been crying. I sat next to her, trying to ease her worries. "Mom, we're not supposed to be worrying about this. We need to wait and see what's going to happen," I told her again.

"Lisa, you can't expect us not to worry. It's hard, you know. I'm just trying to read what I can," she replied.

"I know, but let's just try." I got up from the couch and went to take another bath. It was time to get ready for the CAT scan.

My dad was cooking breakfast, but as usual, I wasn't hungry. I don't think anybody was. My parents didn't go to my CAT scan. I wondered if they really wanted to go but didn't because Wesley and Bev were both going. Bev and her middle son, Sheyne, were there when we pulled up. She brought me a guardian angel pin. I immediately pinned it to the shirt I was wearing, even though I would have to take it off for the test. I knew what it was intended for, and I needed all of the comfort I could get.

When I told the receptionist my name and my appointment

time, she asked if I had finished drinking all of the barium. I was supposed to drink it this morning before I went, but nobody at Dr. McCabe's office had informed me of that. She told me that they would only do an upper-body scan today and give me some barium to drink before my lower-body CAT scan tomorrow morning. Already, things were seeming more complicated, and they got worse when the technician came out to the lobby to give me a large cup of that stuff they call "barium." It looked like a vanilla milkshake, but it tasted like chalk. It wasn't a small, complimentary size cup either. It was as big as they come, and it took all I had in me to drink the entire cup. I was relieved to be able to hold it down. Just then, the same technician came back out with another full cup for me to drink. I truly wanted to cry. I couldn't bear another cup full of that thick, cold, chalky fluid, but somehow I managed to drink it. I started to gag at one point, feeling like I was going to throw up, when a stranger in the lobby warned me that if I did vomit the barium, I would have to drink two full cups all over again. I kept it all down.

After I finished the second cup, the technician came back out to get me. She led me to a small room and instructed me to change into the gown provided. I took everything off, except my socks. Once I finished changing, she took me into the room where I would have the CAT scan.

"Have you ever had a CAT scan before?" she asked.

"No," I answered.

"Well, go ahead and lie down here on the table, with your head on this pillow," she instructed.

I lay down and immediately began shaking and feeling cold, just like I had the day before while waiting for Dr. McCabe to tell me what my X-rays had revealed. I just kept thinking it was all a dream, and I would soon wake up. As I waited for the machine to take pictures of my insides, pictures that would show more than the X-rays had, I questioned whether or not I really even wanted to know what they would reveal. All of these tests were being done to figure out how sick I was. The tests wouldn't reveal that I wasn't sick at all.

"I'm having these tests done because my doctor thinks I have Hodgkin's disease. He says it's a very treatable form of cancer," I told the woman, feeling like I needed to explain why I was there.

"I've heard that it is. Let's just get these done, so you can know for sure," she replied with a warm smile.

"Okay," I agreed.

"Now, are you allergic to iodine?" she asked.

"Not that I know of. I'm not allergic to anything. Why?"

"Because we will be starting an IV in your arm, then injecting iodine in the IV. The iodine helps give contrast to the pictures we'll be taking, along with the barium you drank earlier. The doctor will be with us in a moment to start the IV."

"Good luck finding a vein to use. It took Dr. McCabe's nurse quite a while. She had to warm up my arm and use some type of gel to get the vein to rise enough."

"Well, the doctor is very good. It'll hopefully go better this time. When the iodine is injected, you will notice a metallic taste in your mouth, and your body will start to feel warm for a moment. If you notice anything more than that, just let me know. Okay?"

"Okay. But what else could I feel?"

"Some people, who are allergic to iodine, experience other side effects, but it's unlikely that you will experience those effects."

"Okay."

"Once I start the iodine, the machine will begin taking pictures for about ten minutes. It will tell you when to breathe in and out, to hold your breath, and so on. Follow along, and if you need anything, let me know. I'll be in that small room, but I'll be able to hear and see you."

I kind of laughed to myself when she asked me to follow along. It sounded like I was in school, being asked by my reading teacher to follow along in my book, while the students took turns reading. It made me wish I were sitting in class doing that very thing. Anything other than trying to find out how sick I was.

The doctor walked in and introduced himself, but I quickly forgot his name. He did have a hard time finding a good vein to use, but once he did, he had no problem getting the needle in the right place. I was grateful. He left as quickly as he had entered.

When the iodine entered my body and the warmth she described began at the top of my head, I began to get frightened of what else I might experience as a side effect. The warmth went down my entire body and caused me to sweat. The sensation ended within a few minutes. The anxiety I felt over what might happen to me from the contrast they put in my veins to get a more clear picture of my insides was worse than what I actually experienced. The entire process took about an hour. Wesley, Bev and Sheyne waited in the lobby for me. When I finished, the technician gave me a powdered substance to drink with water in the morning before my lower-body CAT scan. She thought it might be easier for me to drink than the thicker version of the barium. It was worth a try.

As I walked away, the receptionist said, "Be sure to follow the instructions, and don't eat before you come in." I nodded.

"Let's get out of here," I told the three of them. I was very uncomfortable in the jeans I had worn. I was still itching like crazy. The only thing that helped was a bath or a shower. Nothing completely relieved the itching.

"Are you coming over?" I asked Bev and Sheyne, hoping they'd say yes. Her presence has always been comforting to me. We needed to have visitors to entertain, so as not to entertain our worst thoughts.

"Yeah, we'll follow you there."

The first test was over, and I had no idea how many more there would be. I was managing by taking it one appointment at a time.

When we arrived home, things seemed a bit less somber than when we had left earlier. Sheyne started playing with my dad's Labrador, Kizzy, while Bev and my parents talked about the rest of her family. I think Kizzy can sense something is wrong. She is my dad's genius bird dog, and she has been in this family almost as long as I have. That's long enough to sense when things are not right. It seemed like we were successfully not letting ourselves get too worried and upset. The mood soon changed when the phone rang. It was for me.

"Lisa, Dr. McCabe has you scheduled for a biopsy tomorrow. Dr. Malik will be doing the procedure. Is 1:00 P.M. going to be okay for you?" the woman from the hospital asked.

"Yes. I have a lower-body CAT scan in the morning, but I'll be able to be there by 1:00 P.M." I was still taking it one appointment at a time.

"Okay. You'll need to be sure you don't eat anything before you come. You will be under a local anesthetic."

I hung up the phone and told my family about my appointment. "I have a biopsy tomorrow after my CAT scan. It'll just be a local. Dr. McCabe arranged for Dr. Malik to do it, so that's good."

"Dr. Malik is good. We can trust him," Wesley replied.

"Dr. McCabe arranged the biopsy quickly. That's good," my dad added.

"Yeah. That's good. I'm going to take a bath. I just can't stand the itching," I said as I walked toward my bedroom.

I had been dressed for quite a while by then, and I was itching profusely. I found my mom's thin, flannel robe with pink and white stripes and headed for the hall bathroom. I didn't bother grabbing undergarments, as they were too uncomfortable to wear. I shut the door behind me, and then Wesley knocked as I began to undress. I let him in.

"Are you all right?" he asked.

"I'm just tired. I just want to get on with this," I answered, feeling overwhelmed by all of the tests and knowing more would follow.

"Tomorrow will answer everything for us, Lisa."

"I know. I just need another bath. I'm still itching, and I want to relax. Please tell Bev I'll be out in a little while, and ask her not to leave," he kissed my forehead and shut the door behind him.

I turned toward the mirror and looked at myself for a long time, thinking about all that had been happening to me. The eyes that stared back at me seemed not to be my own. Nothing before me seemed to belong, especially the lump that was obvious to me now. I didn't touch it. I just looked in the mirror and into my own eyes, then cried. I hadn't asked why yet, and I wasn't about to. Who was there to ask? God was not to blame. If I could blame God, then I could blame myself. It was best for me to think about tomorrow and know that my questions would be answered after the biopsy.

After I finished my bath, I returned to the kitchen where everyone was waiting for me to begin breakfast. My dad had cooked again, but I still wasn't hungry. I sat with everyone and appeared to eat a few bites, but I really just moved the food from one spot on my plate to another. It wasn't long before the phone rang again. This time it was for my dad. He took the call outside and didn't return to the kitchen for a long time. When he came back inside, his eyes were recognizably red and swollen. My dad had been crying again.

"That was Dr. McCabe on the phone," he announced as he hung up the phone and walked toward the living room, where we had reconvened after finishing breakfast.

"What did he say?" my mom asked.

"He just called to confirm the biopsy for tomorrow and to make sure we were all doing okay. He wanted us to know that he is almost certain this is Hodgkin's disease, and he doesn't want us to be thinking the worst. He said again that if you have to have cancer, then this is the best kind to have," my dad explained with bright eyes. Through the pain I saw the hope that Dr. McCabe had offered him in the phone call.

My dad has always been a man who moves cautiously in the relationships he creates outside of his family and friends. He's a trusting man when given the chance to trust. He knew that Dr. McCabe had always given us that—reasons to trust him.

"You are going to be fine. He's confident of that. He wants us to go to his office after the biopsy tomorrow."

"What for?" I asked.

"I guess just to go over things with us," my dad answered.

"I still have a CAT scan of my lower body tomorrow, don't I?"

"Yes, but that's before the biopsy, so we'll go to his office after the biopsy," he explained.

My dad went back to the phone and made a phone call. When he returned for a second time, I could see that he had been crying again. "I just got off the phone with my mom. I told her Dr. McCabe called. She's real glad he thinks it's treatable. I just know everything is going to be fine. You're going to be fine, Lisa," he said, trying to reassure me again.

"Why were you crying?" I asked, wondering if there was more he had not told me.

"Because Lisa, this is hard. I'm just so glad you're going to be all right. You've got the kind we can beat."

Beverly and Sheyne left soon after, but she will be at my CAT scan and biopsy tomorrow. It's been such a long day. Everyone who knows about this has called today. The phone has been ringing nonstop. I finally went into my parents' room, taking all of my phone calls from there while I rested.

Earlier, we went to get a pizza and to the grocery store, where we ran into Dr. McCabe. It seems funny to me that I have never seen him anywhere other than in his office, until tonight. He said he would see us in his office tomorrow and then said, "Hang in there, kiddo." I'm trying.

I feel so strange tonight. It's all getting foggier to me. I keep hearing all of the people around me saying that they are hoping I have one of the most treatable forms of cancer, but it doesn't seem like all of this could possibly be about me. I tell myself I can get through it, and when I think of it, I ask God to help me.

Most people probably think a person in my position would be praying constantly right now—praying everything is all right inside of me, praying I'll be okay, but I just don't have the strength to do it—to pray for myself. It's like the worst dream I've ever had, and I'm bound to wake up at any minute. I ask for strength and it seems to come, but I just keep asking myself if any of this can possibly be real. As I write these words tonight, I am overcome by the reality of my agony. And that's what it is—true agony. I don't know how I got here. How did I get from one end of my life to the other in just one moment in time? How did everything change so quickly, leaving me in the darkest place of all of my life? I feel empty inside tonight. Like something inside of me has broken, and nobody can fix it. While the others pray for Hodgkin's as the best possible outcome after seeing my X-ray, I realize how very sad it is that at twenty-four years old, the best that I can hope for is the best kind of cancer.

Thursday, December 28

11:54 P.M.—Everyone is in bed. I had to take another bath, because I can't stop itching. It's almost midnight. This day is almost over. I know that when I think back on this day, it will always be remembered as one of the worst of my life. My life; I don't even know how long I will have it.

I had my CAT scan this morning, then waited to have my biopsy. My parents and Wesley were there with me.

When I arrived at The Imaging Center for my test this morning, everything was ready for me. The receptionist gave me one more cup of barium to drink. The same woman who did my CAT scan yesterday met me out in the lobby. I asked her for the trash can because I felt like I was going to throw up. I fought the urge, knowing I would just have to drink the barium all over again. After I finished drinking the thick, disgusting, white chalk, she led me into the room for my second test. She told me I wouldn't have an IV this time, because the doctor felt I would be getting poked enough, and they were just trying to get a basic idea from the pictures today. I was relieved.

My parents seemed to be holding up. When I went into the living room this morning my dad was waiting for me. He asked me to sit down with him.

"I woke up last night, Lisa, out of a deep sleep. I looked at the clock, and it was 11:45 P.M. I don't know what made me look at the clock, but I do know it was at that moment, when I woke up, I realized you're going to be okay. You're going to beat this," he began explaining.

"I know, Dad. That's what you keep telling me," I responded.

"No, Lisa. This is different. Something woke me up and told me you are going to survive. I have worked it out with God. I believe it with every part of my being. You're going to outlive me."

I didn't say anything. I looked at him as he spoke again and could hear the conviction in his words. He really believed what he was telling me.

"There's a picture of you that used to hang in the hallway.

You're at one of my softball games, wearing sunglasses too big for your face. You have a cocky grin on your face, like you are bigger and better than the world."

"Dad!" I said with embarrassment, wondering where this was going.

"No, I mean it, Lisa. You looked like that. That's the look I want to see on your face. That's what will help get you through this. You have to find that attitude again. Like you are bigger, tougher and smarter than this thing. Like you are going to beat it, no matter how hard it gets for you. That's the Lisa I want to see—my ten-year-old, with the cocky grin that says she can conquer the world. We're all here for you, Lisa. You won't go through it alone. That's all I have to say about it. Now give me a hug," he finished as he reached his arms out to me.

I hugged him, but I still did not say anything. I realized that I wasn't supposed to have a reply. I was just supposed to do what he said and find the part of myself he spoke of.

I waited to have my biopsy for over an hour. I had an IV in my arm, even though they said I would only have a local anesthetic. The nurse told me it was just precautionary and to make sure I had enough fluids. I also had a little cap attached to my finger. It monitored my heart rate. I finally asked her to turn down the volume on the monitor, because it was bothering me. She kept asking me if I was nervous, because my heart rate was rather fast, but I honestly didn't feel nervous. My heart had been racing for two days. I guess that was to be expected.

I explained to the nurse why I was there. She told me about a friend of hers who had a swollen lymph node, and it turned out to be nothing. I wasn't holding the same hope, because I already knew. I felt it in my chest when I lifted my arms for the X-ray. I knew.

The biopsy was over at 2:40 P.M. They asked me to stay an

extra thirty minutes to make sure I was all right after the local anesthetic. Wesley stayed with me. My parents went to get us something to eat. They were still trying to feed me, but I wasn't hungry. I don't think they were either. They were just trying to keep themselves busy.

I felt all right after the biopsy. I was glad the lump was gone. Dr. Malik remembered me, after removing my gallbladder two years ago. He used kid gloves with me, per Dr. McCabe's request, I was sure. It only hurt when the large needle penetrated my neck to numb the area they had to cut. They also put oxygen tubes in my nose. That was actually more uncomfortable than the needle.

As the doctor began to cut along the right side of my collarbone, I felt compelled to make one request. "When you take it out, I want to see it," I told him.

I could tell he and the others were shocked by what I'd said. "You want me to show the lymph node to you?" he asked, making sure he had heard me correctly.

"Yes. I want to see it when you take it out. I want to see what it looks like," I answered.

"Well, all right," he reluctantly complied.

"I want to see what is about to change my life." As I said those words, I noticed one of the nurses looking away from me, then down at the floor. I think it made her sad to hear me say that, but I meant it. When my grandpa was dying of cancer, I always wondered what it looked like—the stuff inside of him called cancer, consuming him and invading every part of his body.

It didn't take long for Dr. Malik to cut out the swollen node, and when he did nobody said a word. None of them said everything looked fine, or it was probably nothing. I think at that moment everyone knew. "Okay Lisa, we've got it out," Dr. Malik said as he held the lymph node in front of me to see. It was about the size of a golf ball and had tissue and blood all around it. It was just a solid mass of tissue from what I could see. It was what is on the inside of my body that we were all waiting to find out more about.

"Okay. I've seen it," I said as I turned my head away. "Are you giving me stitches?"

"No, Dr. McCabe doesn't want you all scarred up, so we are going to tape you up real tight. Just leave the bandages on for at least five days, all right?"

"All right. Thank you, Dr. Malik."

"Oh you're welcome, Lisa. We'll send this to the lab and have the results as soon as possible," he explained.

"Dr. McCabe asked me to go by his office after we are finished here," I said, wondering if Dr. Malik knew why.

"Then go ahead and do that. You only had a local, but you might still be tired and groggy, so just be sure to drink lots of fluids and get some rest," he instructed.

And with that, he left the room. The whole thing only took about twenty minutes. I was glad to see Wesley waiting in the lobby for me when I came out. He didn't want to leave with my parents, in case I got out before they returned. We went to Dr. McCabe's office after the biopsy. It was only around the corner. I wasn't sure what the purpose of our visit was, but I was ready to do what he asked.

We were ushered to the back lobby to wait for Dr. McCabe. Beverly and Sheyne waited outside for us. It seemed very unusual for the nurse to put us in the back hallway.

She didn't make us wait at all, because they wanted me to sit down in a comfortable place, knowing I had just come from surgery.

"Why are we here?" I asked Linda, the nurse.

"Because the doctor wants you to find out the results of the biopsy today," she explained.

"But the tests aren't already done, are they?" I asked, looking very confused.

"Well, this will be a preliminary diagnosis, because we don't want you to have to wait. This way you won't have to worry all weekend about the results."

"This is good. Now we'll know," my dad agreed.

We waited for Dr. McCabe to come around the corner.

"Hey kiddo. How'd it go?" he asked as he shook hands with my dad and Wesley, then hugged my mom.

"All right. They only taped me up tight. Thanks."

"Less scarring that way. I'm going to make a phone call and see if we can't find something out for you," he said as he walked back around the corner.

There I was, sitting in the same place I had sat just two days before. I heard him get on the phone.

"This is Dr. McCabe. Dr. Malik just did a lymph biopsy for me on Lisa Brawley. They should have taken a look at it by now. I'm waiting on a preliminary . . . No, I'll hold," he said.

I sat there shaking from head to toe again. "Are you cold?" my mom asked.

"No, just scared," I answered.

"I told you everything is going to be all right. It's Hodgkin's, Lisa. They can treat that. I know it's Hodgkin's," my dad said, trying to comfort me and probably himself as well. Wesley held my hand tighter.

While waiting for the diagnosis, I don't know if the thought of having Hodgkin's disease gave me any comfort. The thought of having any kind of cancer growing recklessly inside of my body scared me to the very core of my being.

"I love you," Wesley said, holding my hand even tighter.

"I love you," I told him as tears began to well up in my eyes.

I heard Dr. McCabe thank the person on the phone. I don't know what he had previously arranged or what strings had been pulled, but it was done. As he came around the corner again, I could feel every muscle in my body tighten. I held on to Wesley with both hands, bracing myself for what would come next. Dr. McCabe began walking toward me.

"Lisa, it's Hodgkin's."

When I heard him say the word, I let go of Wesley's hand, and I believe a part of myself as well. It had been confirmed. I had cancer, and what was left of my innocence was lost— the innocence of believing that nothing like this could ever happen to me. I felt like bursting into tears, but I could not. Just one single tear fell from my cheek to my hand, once again holding Wesley's.

"This is good, right? This is what it had to be, right?" my dad asked the doctor.

"Yes. Lisa, if you have to get one, this is the one to get," my doctor explained.

My mom had tears in her eyes. My parents walked toward me, both hugging me at the same time.

"But . . . But . . ." I tried to speak, but I could not.

"We're going to get you well, Lisa. We're going to get through this together," my mom said as she hugged me even tighter.

"I'll take care of you," Wesley added. "We'll all take care of you."

I tried to speak again, but I still could not say anything.

"You understand this is the best possible thing that could have come from this. I wish it had been nothing. I wish I could have sent you home with antibiotics and your swollen glands, but that's not what this is. This is treatable. Hodgkin's disease responds very well to treatment," Dr. McCabe explained. "We'll still have to run more tests to find out what stage we are dealing with, but you'll have chemo and then some radiation."

"Will she have any more surgery?" my mom asked.

"No. There won't be any more surgery with this type of cancer," he continued.

Cancer. It was the first time he had even used that word when speaking to me, but that's what it is. Call it Hodgkin's disease; call it whatever you want. It's still cancer. I'm only twenty-four years old, have only been married for two years, have never given birth to a child, haven't graduated from college, and I have cancer.

We followed Dr. McCabe to the front desk, where he gave me a card with the name of the oncologist I would be seeing. Up until that point, it had never even occurred to me that another doctor would be treating me. The oncologist's name was Dr. Verma, and I was scheduled to see him on Tuesday, January 2.

Wesley and my dad had already gone outside to tell Beverly and Sheyne the news. My mom stayed inside with me until the appointment scheduling was complete.

"You'll be seeing Dr. Verma on a regular basis, but you can come and see me any time you like in between. I definitely want to see you back here in a month. Don't worry. You're in good hands. I was the first one to hold you in my arms, don't you remember?" Dr. McCabe asked with a smile as he hugged me good-bye.

"I remember," my mom softly whispered. "I remember."

As I walked out the door of his office for the second time in only two days and realized a rare occurrence had just taken place, I was grateful for having been told my fate today, rather than next week. I tried to find the good in what had just happened, but all I could feel was despair.

Beverly hugged me when I got outside. "You doing okay?" she asked with concern.

"I guess so. I just want to go home. Are you guys coming?"

"Of course. We'll meet you there." Bev knew I needed a full house.

While Wesley drove me home, I asked him, "Are you scared?"

"No. I know now that you will be okay. You are going to get well," he reassured me.

"Do you really believe that?" I questioned him again.

"With everything inside of me, Lisa. We'll all get you through it. We'll do it together," he answered as he kissed my hand twice.

I leaned my head against the cold car window and said quietly to myself, "I'm counting on it."

Four

Tuesday, January 2, 1996

The New Year has come and gone. It was uneventful; we all stayed home. Wesley went to bed at 10:30 P.M., and my dad went to bed soon after that. My mom stayed up with me.

When I removed the bandages from my lymph node biopsy this morning, I immediately began to cry, horrified by what I saw. I expected to see a thin cut about an inch long. Instead, I saw a swollen, bright purple cut that was more than two inches long. I ran out of the bathroom looking for Wesley. I found him getting out of the shower.

"What is it? What's wrong?" Wesley said trying to wrap a towel around himself and get to me at the same time.

"Look!" I cried, showing him what I had discovered. "It's huge. They said it would be minor. This is *not* minor!"

"Lisa, it will fade. It doesn't look as bad as you think."

By then, we'd made our way to the bedroom, but in a fit of panic I left him there and went to the kitchen to find my parents. I entered crying and showed my mom the impending scar. My dad was talking on the telephone when he heard me crying.

"I've got to go. Something is happening here," he said as he abruptly hung up the phone.

Wesley soon entered the kitchen. They all tried to convince me that the scar would heal and be minimal once the swelling went down.

I think I was crying because I was angry. I cried for having a cut in such a visible place that would always have to be explained to those who noticed and asked about it. It just seems unfair to me that I will have such a vivid reminder in a place that I will see almost every time I look into a mirror. As if watching my hair fall out is not going to be hard enough—at least the hair loss will be temporary.

I am having a difficult time getting rest during the day. I am often tired, but I have been saving my sleep for nighttime. I have to be sure I am tired when things quiet down and the others are ready for bed.

A few nights ago, I started feeling some anxiety about staying up while everyone was asleep, so I made a simple request. I asked that one of them stay up with me until I am tired enough to go to sleep. They agreed to do that for me.

I usually get up at least three times during the night, sometimes to take a bath to relieve the itching, other times just because the pressure in my chest makes sleeping difficult. When I lay on my back, it feels like I have a balloon in my chest and my breathing is labored. When I lay on my stomach, I feel like I am suffocating. I am always afraid that if I fall asleep in that position I will stop breathing in my sleep, so I am training myself to sleep on my left side. My heart doesn't beat as fast that way.

My dad's sister Joyce, and my cousins Darla and Nicole, came to visit us this weekend. They brought chicken enchiladas. They were asking me a lot of questions, and I felt comfortable answering them. I don't mind talking about it. It seems that's all we have been talking about since last Tuesday.

My aunt said that she had some mosquito bites that itched badly and made her think of how badly I have been suffering with this merciless itching. I showed them my legs and the bottom of my feet. I had to clip the skin away from my feet again, because I had scratched them so much that small pieces of skin began to tear and bleed. My feet still bleed sometimes, but I can't stop scratching. They aren't even ticklish anymore.

Today I go to see Dr. Verma. I learned over the weekend that an oncologist is a doctor who oversees chemotherapy treatments. He'll be helping me decide which type of treatment I will take. Wesley and my parents will go with me. Dr. Verma is supposed to have the results back from the CAT scans.

I told my parents that I think it's probably in my lower body, although I don't have any idea what that means, other than what Dr. McCabe told me the first day, "It's easily treated, especially if only found above the diaphragm." At this point, I can't see how it makes any difference. Whether or not it's in my chest or anywhere else doesn't really matter to me. It's here. That won't change.

11:52 P.M.—As I lay flat on my back, I realize that the days just keep getting more difficult to bear. Our meeting with Dr. Verma was both informative and overwhelming. We had to wait quite a while to see him. Carrie, Dr. Verma's receptionist, said that he was trying to clear out the office so he would be able to give us as much time as we needed with him. That put me at ease. I was glad to know he was getting ready for our first appointment. I know Dr. McCabe will keep me in capable hands.

While we waited in the lobby, I paid attention again to the people who came in and out of the office and wondered why each of them were there. None of them looked like they had cancer. They all had their hair. It just goes to show that you never know who is well and who is not. Cancer is so silent. It's silent until it confuses a body enough to let out a roar, and with that roar, the one hope is that it's not too late.

Dr. Verma discussed the statistics involved with Hodgkin's disease patients and the likeliness of a fifteen-year survival rate. With the treatments they are using today, I have about an 85 percent chance of remission. That number is somewhat comforting, but I am constantly aware of the reality the other side of that statistic holds. I realize I am now a number and where I will fall among this statistic is anyone's guess. No one can tell me for sure, except my dad, but he is speaking by faith and his will for me to survive. When I am feeling weak, I listen to the statistics. And when I cannot find solace in the statistics, I listen to my dad and to Wesley.

I was coping with the conversation as well as could be expected until the subject of risks from chemotherapy came up. It never occurred to me that I could choose not to have chemotherapy, but Dr. Verma felt certain that I would better benefit from the combination of both chemotherapy and radiation therapy.

"Radiation therapy is hard on the heart and can cause long-term damage to the arteries. It can cause them to harden. If you were to have only radiation, I feel your chances of remission would be lessened drastically. We would have to administer far too much radiation for the amount of cancer that is in your chest. The CAT scans do not show any lower body involvement, but we will have to run some more tests to be sure. Chemotherapy also has its risks, but each of them are lessened when we do not do too much of one or the other. You are a young girl, and we want to put the least amount of strain on your body as possible, so that if we are able to get rid of the cancer with these treatments, you will have a healthy body to carry you through the rest of your life."

"I am just afraid of all the things I have heard about chemotherapy. I can deal with my hair falling out, but what if something else goes really wrong?" I asked him.

"That's why I am here. It's my job to regulate your chemotherapy treatments. I will make sure that your blood counts are at a stable enough level to continue treatment as scheduled, although in some cases there may be delays in your treatment program," he continued.

"What kind of delays?" my mother asked.

"If your daughter's blood counts are too low for treatment, we usually wait an extra week before continuing. Some problems can be managed with new drugs that are available to bring up the white and red blood cell counts, but other blood counts have to be waited out. Now there are some other risks involved over a long-term basis."

"What other risks?" my dad asked. He was sitting with my mom across from Wesley and me. Dr. Verma was sitting at the head of the table.

"Lisa's blood cells are made in the bone marrow, and because the bone marrow is affected by the chemotherapy and radiation, there is a small risk of her developing leukemia even if she recovers from Hodgkin's disease."

I felt so overwhelmed as he continued to explain the long-term risks. I felt like crying. But just as before, the tears did not surface. I covered my face with my hands and began to sink in my chair. "You mean even if I survive this cancer, I could end up with something worse later in my life?" I asked.

"It's a small risk, only about 3 to 6 percent, but I want you to be aware of these risks, enabling you to make an informed decision." Dr. Verma tried to comfort me, but I knew he sensed the despair in all of us as we continued asking questions about my uncertain fate.

"What else?" Wesley proceeded.

Could any of us bear to hear more? Could any of us walk out of that office the same people, after already being changed by last week's diagnosis? I thought that it couldn't possibly get any worse, but it did. With every word the doctor spoke, it got worse.

"There is a risk of second tumors from radiation therapy, but again, these risks are better than the alternative," Dr. Verma continued with caution.

"How much risk?" I asked.

"About 18 percent," he answered.

"But with this treatment program, it is likely that Lisa will get through the treatment, survive the cancer and go on to live a healthy and normal life?" my dad asked, always the optimist.

"Yes, there is a very good chance of this, but there is one more thing I need to discuss with you. If we do not find any cancer below the diaphragm in further testing then that means we are dealing with stage II of this disease. The protocol for this staging of Hodgkin's disease is administering ABVD through an IV every two weeks. ABVD stands for Adriamycin, Bleomycin, Velban and DTIC. Then, you would continue with radiation therapy. The amount of radiation therapy you would receive will depend largely on how your body responds to chemotherapy. You would have anywhere from three to six cycles of ABVD, each being given on day one and day fifteen of your treatment schedule. You must also be aware that there have been cases of infertility among patients after receiving this type of chemotherapy."

I'd had all I could take. I told myself it was over. There was no use in fighting this thing. It already had me. In just one week, it had taken my life and turned it into something that

I could barely manage to participate in. It had taken away the part of me that enabled me to be enough of a woman to create and give life to another human being. I would have to withdraw from school until I was better, if I got better, and it had the three most important people in my life looking like they wanted to die themselves.

I looked at Wesley when Dr. Verma told us about the possibility of infertility. I saw the tears well up in his eyes. My mother was crying quiet tears at that point, but my father just kept looking as strong as he could. I felt so sorry for them all, more sorry for them than I did myself. My dad had told me just days before that he was certain I would survive and that I had to believe it, too. I think when he made that pact with God, he was completely unaware of what I would be up against. In that pact with God, did my dad know we would face the risk of me never having a child of my own?

"Now the risk is slight. Certain types of chemotherapy affect fertility among men more than they do women, but there is still a risk. Your chances of having a child would be lessened if you had lower body radiation, but as long as we do not find any other involvement in further tests, your chances of having children will be much greater. In any event, I advise you to consider the option of freezing some of your eggs for later fertilization. I can recommend a doctor in the area who specializes in this."

None of us uttered a word after that. He asked us if we had further questions about treatment, then he gave us some pamphlets to take home about Hodgkin's disease and treatment options. The treatable cancer, Hodgkin's disease, hardly even came up in that hour and a half consultation. It was during the discussion that I realized we were up against something bigger than we first thought. It was getting more and more complicated. More tests, more doctors, but still no guarantees.

"I am going to schedule a bone marrow biopsy for you, as well as a gallium scan."

"What are those?" I dared to ask.

"They'll take a sample of your bone marrow, generally from your hips, then they'll test the sample to make sure there is not any cancer involvement in the marrow. The gallium scan is used to get detailed pictures of your soft tissue, namely your lymph nodes. We'll be able to see from that test whether or not there is any cancer in your lower body. This test is the best available to find out exactly what stage of the disease we are dealing with."

"Is the bone marrow biopsy painful?" I asked.

"You will feel discomfort and pressure, but the doctors are very skilled in this procedure. They will numb the area with a local anesthetic before they begin."

He told me to go home and wait for a call about the bone marrow biopsy. He was hoping I would be able to get the test done later in the day. Just when I thought the worst of the day was over, I naively went to my bone marrow biopsy, only to discover my body had truly betrayed me.

Wesley and I arrived at the hospital and waited for at least twenty minutes. Eventually, I was led through several doors and to a room that had in it a hospital bed and several people in white lab coats preparing for the procedure. I had asked if Wesley could come with me, but the nurse told me they would send for him after the procedure.

I had on my usual attire since the itching started months ago, sweats and a T-shirt to help make me comfortable. I didn't have to change into one of their fancy robes for the biopsy.

"Now Lisa, go ahead and get up on the table and lay on your stomach," the only man in the room instructed. "Have they told you anything about how the biopsy is done?"

"Not really. My doctor just said that you would be getting

marrow from my hips and testing it to make sure there is not any cancer involvement. Is it going to be painful?" I asked.

"Well, you will feel some pressure, but we will numb the area before we begin," he said, confirming Dr. Verma's description of the pain level I might experience.

One of the nurses was busy getting an IV started for me. She did pretty well. Everyone in the room seemed very kind. They had "MD Anderson Cancer Center" patches on the front of their jackets.

"You guys are from MD Anderson in Houston?" I asked them.

"Yes. Are you familiar with that hospital?" the doctor replied.

"Yeah, a lady I used to work for went through treatment there for breast cancer."

"How is she doing?" the doctor asked.

"She died."

"Oh . . . well, I am sorry to hear that," he stumbled in his reply.

"She only had good things to say about your hospital. The type of breast cancer she had kept reappearing, and finally, after five years of battling it, she died."

"Well, we're going to try and get you fixed up and through this as simply as possible," he added, changing the subject. "You're a pretty popular girl in this town. Everyone is talking about Dr. McCabe's lifelong patient," he explained.

"Why? Because I have cancer?"

"No, because he says you're quite a kid with quite a family."

I lay on my stomach as they lowered my sweatpants below my hips and began explaining the steps of the procedure. I looked to my right and, in the reflection of the computer screen above the bed, I caught a glimpse of the needle they'd be using. The needle was at least six inches long. I'd never been afraid of needles, until then. The doctor and nurses had been very careful to conceal the tools. No wonder.

"I can see that needle reflecting on the blank screen above my head," I informed them.

"Put this towel over the screen," the doctor instructed a nurse. After she covered it up, he asked me, "Can you see anything now?"

"No. It's fine now," I answered.

I was given an IV for Demerol to be administered for pain during the biopsy. When the nurse finished inserting the IV, the doctor explained the procedure before he began. "I am going to insert a small needle into your left hip. This is a local anesthetic and will numb the area before I begin to retrieve the bone marrow."

"What is bone marrow?"

"It's the place inside of your bones where blood cells are made. Like white blood cells that fight infection and other vital cells that are constantly being produced in your bone marrow," he explained.

"How do you retrieve the bone marrow?" I asked.

"After the area is numb, I'll insert another type of needle that will penetrate the bone and will withdraw marrow from inside your hip. I'll do it as quickly as possible, but you must try and remain still," he explained.

By then, he had inserted the needle and began tapping the needle's tip on my hipbone. It was uncomfortable. "Am I supposed to be able to feel you tapping on my bone?"

"Let's give it a minute to absorb, then we'll check to see if you need another shot."

We waited, then he inserted the needle again.

"I can feel the needle going through my skin."

"Let's give her another dose," he said to the nurse.

He repeated the process and asked, "Can you feel it when I do this?" tapping on my bone again with the needle's tip.

"Not as much as before, but I can still feel it."

The doctor started massaging the area he had injected, trying to make it penetrate deeper. "How about now?"

"That feels better."

"Okay, Lisa, here we go. I am going to start slowly. Tell me if you feel any pain."

I didn't feel him enter my skin, but suddenly I felt something pierce my bone. "I can feel that! I can feel it! It hurts!" I exclaimed.

"Okay. Okay. Lisa, I'm backing out. We'll give you another shot before we go any further."

"Another shot won't help. I couldn't feel it go through my skin. I felt it when you started to go through the bone. Isn't there something more you can do?" I asked him.

"Unfortunately, there is nothing we can do to numb the bone. Let's just give it another try. It's going to hurt, but if you can hang in there, I can finish more quickly and get it over with," he explained.

"Here, Lisa, hold my hand. Squeeze it as hard as you need to," one of the nurses said as she placed her hand in mine.

I could hear the doctor talking softly to the other nurses. He could not figure out why I could still feel the needle and why the local anesthetic wasn't alleviating some of the pain.

"I'm going in again, Lisa. Hold onto her hand and try to let me get in and get it done. I'll go as fast as I can."

I buried my face in the pillow and squeezed the nurse's hand tightly. I could feel the tool enter my bone for the second time as he hovered over the back of me and used the weight of his body to force it into my body. The pressure was excruciating. "Stop! Stop! It hurts! Please stop!" I screamed and pleaded with him.

"Okay, okay. Lisa I'll stop right here, but I'll leave it in. We're almost done. I'm in now; I just need to aspirate the bone marrow. Just take some deep breaths and tell me when you're ready," he compliantly said. I turned my head to look at him. Sweat was pouring down his face.

I waited a few moments, then told him, "Go ahead. Just please hurry."

"You're doing great, Lisa. You're doing great. Just a few minutes more," the nurse holding my hand said, trying to comfort me.

I could hear him ask another nurse for the tool that would aspirate the marrow, and then he inserted it into the hole he had made. "Okay, Lisa. You're going to feel this. Try and let me get it out, so I can remove the marrow as fast as I can."

Just then, a shooting pain shot down from the middle of my chest down to my legs. I let out a roar of screams and straightened my body out until it was as straight and stiff as it could be. "Oh, God! Dear God! Please help me! Please help me!"

"Lisa, I've almost got it!"

"Just finish! Just get it out of me! Oh, God, get it out of me!" I screamed.

All of the nurses began talking to me at once. They told me to hang in there and that I was doing well until, finally, he had finished and removed the corkscrew-like instrument from the center of my hip.

The doctor held up a small, clear container filled with a white, cloudy fluid that had streaks of my blood in it. "I got it, Lisa. I got enough," he said.

I could barely see the contents of the cup, but I could see enough to know that it came from somewhere inside of me that he had to dig deep to retrieve it. In his hand, he held more than my bone marrow, he held the core of my being, the core of my body, and again, like the other doctors, he was searching my insides for more cancer.

"Okay, Lisa. You're doing great," he said.

"Yes. You're doing better than most people," a nurse added.

"How can I be doing better than most people?" I questioned. "I've been screaming at the top of my lungs."

"Because most people yell profanity, you've been yelling for God," the nurse holding my hand answered as she brushed my damp hair away from my face.

I took deep breaths and tried to relax. Then the doctor said, "Okay, Lisa. Now we need to do the other side."

He repeated the same procedure as before by inserting three doses of the local anesthetic into my opposite hip. Again, I could feel it, but I didn't say anything until he asked, "Can you still feel it?"

"Not much. Just get it over with," I answered.

When he penetrated the center of my body again, the pain was worse than before. "Oh, God! It's worse! It's worse! Get it out of me! Get it out!" I screamed.

"Just give me a minute, Lisa. Just a few more minutes. I've almost got it. Just a minute more."

"No! Get it out! Get it out now!" I demanded.

"Lisa, I think I've got it. I'm taking it out. I think I've got enough."

I looked at one of the nurses as he held up the clear container again. I saw a look of despair on her face, and then I looked closely at the container. It was practically empty.

"Oh, God, no. Please, can someone go get my husband? Please. I need him in here," I begged of them.

"Lisa, I didn't get enough. I have to go back in. We'll get your husband as soon as we're finished."

"Isn't there enough from the other side?" I asked him.

"We have to get a complete sample from both sides or they'll make us repeat it. As long as they don't find any cancer involved in the marrow and your treatment is successful, you won't ever have to repeat this test again."

"Just do what you have to," I told him.

As he began again, the pain of the corkscrew penetrating

my flesh was as painful as the previous entries. I let out only one plea for God's help. The nurse directly assisting him said sternly, "Don't stop. Just keep going. Get it all this time."

He did, but I had stopped fighting the pain. As much as I wished I could somehow remove myself from my body, I just lay there silently praying for God to rescue me.

"Lisa? Are you with us?" the doctor asked. "You have to stay with us."

I didn't answer him. I was lost. I could find no strength to draw from, and I could find no words to make him feel better about having to chisel through my flesh and into my bones.

"Lisa . . . talk to us," he said.

"What do you want me to say?" I asked him as I lay with my arms limp to my side. I was no longer crying, the pain was beyond evoking anymore tears. Even the screaming had stopped. I just lay before them in emptiness. They continued trying to get me to rejoin them and speak.

"Talk about anything you want," one of the nurses answered.

After a moment of silence, I asked, "Do you want to hear about how I met my husband?"

"Yes. Tell us about that," the doctor answered.

"I was eight years old and he was ten. He'd just moved down the street from me. He had been living with his mom, Donna, and stepdad, Jimbo, in Texas before moving to California to live with his dad and his stepmom, Laverne. The day he arrived, he befriended my brother and all of the neighborhood boys. They were playing football in my front yard. I was inside with one of my friends, so we decided to go outside to see about the new guy," I began. "When I opened the door and stepped out onto the front porch, I saw him at the top of a pile of other boys. He stopped and looked at me longer than an uninterested boy would have and smiled. I smiled back. He was wearing corduroy pants, the color of red brick, and his shirt had the same colored stripes. His hair was beyond blond. It was white and long enough to brush against his shoulders. His face was covered in faint freckles and even though I didn't like freckles, I liked him. Before he even uttered a word, his fate had been sealed."

"You remember all of that from when you were only eight years old?" one of the nurses asked. I didn't answer her. I just kept telling my story, because even though I was telling it more for myself than for them, it seemed to lessen the pain and if that was the only way I could bring his comfort into the room, I wanted to keep talking. By then, I was feeling the effects of the Demerol.

"He lived in California with his dad for two years until they all moved back to Texas. He was the object of my affection throughout both years, but I was hardly the object of his. He considered me more of a pest, especially since he and my brother had become best friends, and my brother and I never got along.

"For some reason, I don't remember the day he moved away for good. His whole family packed up a utility trailer and drove as far as Sacramento, when his dad turned the car around and drove back to Redding to give it one more try for his wife's sake. She wanted to live near her family, but soon after, they left again, passed the Sacramento sign and kept on going.

"I finally saw Wesley again five years later when I went to Texas to spend Thanksgiving with his family. He was on leave from the Navy, and I believe I fell in love with him during that visit. Wesley finally noticed me, but he was turning eighteen and was now a man who was in the Navy, and I was still a fifteen-year-old kid who had to answer to her parents. I always told my friends that when I was old enough to get on a plane and go visit him I would, and if he didn't fall in love with me in a weekend, I would forget about him. So when I was old enough, I got on a plane and went to see him. I arrived on a Friday, and he told me he loved me on the following Sunday. We got married three years later."

When I finished speaking, one of the nurses handed a tissue to the nurse who was still holding my hand.

"That's the best story I've ever heard," the crying nurse said as she wiped her eyes. "Where is your husband now?"

"He's out in the lobby. He's waiting for me."

"Go get him. We're all finished here," the doctor said in a voice that hushed his own emotions.

After he gave both containers to the nurse standing to his left, he looked down at me. With his sterile cap drenched in sweat, his hands shaking from the way he had just rattled my spirit, and his eyes resembling a deer's caught in headlights, he spoke to me softly as he placed his hand on my forehead. "Now I know why Dr. McCabe speaks so highly of you. You're the bravest I've met in a long, long time."

He walked to the door, opened it, and then turned to speak to me once again. "You keep fighting this cancer the way you fought it today and you're going to outlive us all." The door closed on its own behind him.

I don't know if the anesthetic had finally taken effect or if speaking of the way Wesley and I began somehow served as the most natural pain reliever I could have had. Maybe once I reached a certain level of pain I could no longer feel anything. Maybe God had again intervened and rescued me from the feeling of complete defeat and carried me out of that room and onto my front porch of sixteen years ago. Whatever happened, I knew it could not erase the torment of what this disease had forced the doctors to search for and the ways in which they had to search to find it. My body had betrayed me. Even if God had rescued my spirit for that moment, I knew more of me had been lost, and I knew I would never be the same.

One nurse remained holding my hand after the other people wearing white lab coats had left the room.

She started to leave when Wesley entered the room, but before she did, she looked at both of us and said quietly, "I asked him to give you more Demerol. He just wouldn't do it. I asked him to." I managed a smile of recognition for her, but there were no words to offer.

Wesley had entered the room smiling, completely unaware of what had just taken place. He, as I had, thought it would just be another routine test. When he saw the look on my pale face, his torrent of tears met mine, and we held each other as we cried for all that had wreaked havoc on our lives. Without words, we cried for the children we may never have, for the joy we may never find again, and, I believe, for the two little kids who saw each other for the first time in my front yard. And we wished with all of our might that we could be them again.

Five

Friday, January 5

I am still a little sore from the biopsy, but the discomfort is lessening. I now know that the only people who described the pain of a bone marrow biopsy with the word "pressure" or "discomfort" never had one.

I had a gallium scan on Wednesday, Thursday and today. It wasn't painful. A nurse injected the gallium fluid into my IV after the bone marrow biopsy, giving the fluid enough time to secrete through my soft tissue before I started the tests on Wednesday.

The first day was the most uncomfortable, because I still had the bandages on my hips from the biopsy. The nurse put them there after the procedure and made me lay on my back for an hour after to make sure my blood properly clotted, so I wouldn't get an infection.

I had to lay still and flat on my back for the gallium scan. A machine was placed centimeters from my body, scanning it and taking three-dimensional pictures of my soft tissue and lymph nodes from every angle. No pain. No "pressure."

During the first day of testing, I could see the screen that showed the insides of my body. I tried not to look at it, because I knew it would show me exactly where and how much cancer there was growing recklessly inside of my body. I was frightened to look, but I felt compelled to see it.

When I looked at the screen, I saw the blackness of my lymph nodes. The skeleton on the screen was my own and the cancer within it also belonged to me. From the top, right side of my chest to the middle of my rib cage, all I could see was darkness.

I kept looking at it, afraid to see what the machine would find as it searched further down my body. Just then, the technician entered the room and asked how I was doing.

"Could you please turn off the screen?" I asked him.

He seemed surprised until he looked at the screen and saw what I had been looking at for the past several minutes. "Oh, sure. That's no problem," he answered.

"I know it's there. I just don't want to see it," I explained.

"I understand," he said as he turned off the screen.

As nice as he was, he didn't understand.

I have an appointment with Dr. Verma next Thursday. By then, he will have the results of my bone marrow biopsy and the gallium scans.

I had a lung test yesterday that simply required me to breathe into a tube a number of times while the machine measured my lung capacity. Dr. Verma said the test is done to have a record of what my lungs were like before chemotherapy and radiation. Then, I'll repeat the test after I have completed both treatments.

I also had an EKG. He wanted to make sure I had a healthy heart before starting treatment, because Adriamycine, one of the chemotherapy drugs I will be taking, and radiation can be hard on the heart.

My heart continues to beat rapidly, but Dr. Verma explained

that it's because of the pressure of the tumors near my heart. He said it would subside once the tumors begin to shrink.

I was scheduled for an appointment with the fertility doctor he referred us to, but my gallium scan ran late, so we missed it. On the way home, Wesley and I discussed making another appointment.

"I know it's important that we are able to have children, but I just don't know that I can walk into one more doctor's office knowing I'll have to go through another procedure. Especially since we've been told it would be painful for them to retrieve the eggs from my ovaries," I explained to Wesley.

"I was thinking the same thing. I didn't want to say anything, but if you feel the same way, then let's just forget about rescheduling an appointment. Let's just get you well and deal with the rest later," he agreed.

"I truly believe that God won't let me go through all of this and then watch us be deprived of having a child. I have to believe that," I told him.

"Well, this is no time to start losing your faith in God, so just keep believing, and when the time is right, we'll have a family."

I unbuckled my seat belt, so I could scoot closer to him in the car. I rested my head on his shoulder. "I love you, Wesley."

"Me, too."

Sunday, January 7

8:30 A.M.—During the past few days, as much as I hated admitting it, I had been thinking about Wesley needing to go back to Texas on our originally scheduled flight. I knew he needed to go and get more of our clothes and whatever else we would need for the rest of our stay. It was obvious that we wouldn't manage on my parents' two cars. We needed to have our own car here.

Wesley was having the same thoughts, but he knew how I would feel about him leaving. We finally talked it over last night.

"I know you don't want me to go right now, but the sooner I go, the sooner I can get back," he said, trying to comfort me.

"But you'll miss my first chemotherapy. I need you here for that."

"Lisa, do you really? I mean, can you get through it with your parents and Bev to help you? If you can't, then I'll stay. I am fully prepared to take care of you every day throughout this, but you know we need our own car. We don't know how long we are going to be here."

"I know having my parents with me would be enough, but you're the one who takes me to all of these appointments and tests. Most of the time, the only thing that gets me through is knowing that you're on the other side of the doors waiting for me."

"And I will be on the other side of those doors waiting for you after I get back. I know you are going through a lot right now. We all are, but do you realize how difficult it is for me to live here with your parents? We are all trying to take care of you, and that's fine, but I think me going back home to get our things will allow me to regroup and prepare myself for what is ahead."

I know that it is hard for Wesley to live with my parents. I have been gone from home so long that it's even hard for me, but we both know this is where we belong right now. Wesley and I have always managed to make it through the difficult times together. We've learned to rely on each other. Because of this, I have learned to rely on my parents less, but when I am in their house, I seem to revert back to my childlike ways of seeking their approval and wanting to please them. It's frustrating for Wesley to watch. I just keep hoping that once treatment begins and we have a better idea of what getting me well will mean, we'll all find our place in the process. For now, we have left school and our jobs in Texas behind, and with both of our families helping, we will be able to remain here as long as necessary.

"How long will you be gone?"

"I don't know. About two weeks."

"That's a long time."

"Four days of that will be traveling. I am not leaving you here to go through this alone. You have your parents here, and I know they are a comfort to you or I wouldn't even consider it. And to tell you the truth, I wouldn't mind getting to spend a little time with my family. I need them, too."

"I know. I just wish none of this were even happening. I wish we could fly home together, go back to school in a few weeks, and everything would be the way it was before."

"So do I. All of us do."

He's leaving this afternoon.

10:58 P.M.—It's late, and I can't sleep. I took Wesley to the Sacramento airport earlier today. Amber, Wesley's youngest sister, rode with us so I wouldn't have to drive back alone. It's a two and a half-hour drive from here. As difficult as it was, I know we did the right thing. He'll call me when he gets to his Uncle Ronnie's house in Dallas and every day after.

On our way there, we talked about my being scared of chemotherapy and of dying of this.

I asked Wesley, "Do you think I am going to be okay, or do you think I might die?"

And quick as a flash, he answered, "I know you are going to be okay. There's no doubt in my mind you're going to be okay."

"You really believe that?"

"I absolutely believe it."

The conviction in his words and the way that he offered

them made me cry. I felt badly for Amber having to listen to us. I knew it must have been hard for her. She's the person I have known the longest in my life. Of course I have known my parents, my brother and other people in my family longer, but I have known her all of her life. I remember when her mother, Laverne, was pregnant with her and always wore a plaid robe while she was on bed rest. I knew her before she was even born.

She's grown up a lot since their dad died in October of 1994. I respect her for her strength and for handling the events in her life with such maturity.

I apologized to her for starting to cry. "I am sorry you have to see this and listen to us talk about it."

"You don't have to apologize," she said.

"I know, but I just don't usually cry about it," I explained.

And in her innocent wisdom that I admire, she replied, "Well, maybe you should."

Thursday, January 12

11:10 P.M.—Wesley has been gone for five days now. I miss him. He arrived safely in Dallas on Sunday night and called me as soon as his plane landed. He called me two more times before he went to sleep and again when we woke up in the morning. On Monday night, he went with his Uncle Ronnie to a pool hall and played pool for a few hours. He has kept his promise and still hasn't had a drink since August. The day after this all began, he made the comment that he could sure use a drink, but I replied, "That wouldn't do either one of us any good right now," and it ended there. I can only hope that in the weeks and months ahead, Wesley will draw strength from what he has learned in the months he hasn't been drinking. After his dad died, he drank so often that it threatened to destroy our marriage. At the time, alcohol seemed to be the only remedy to numb his pain. On the night Wesley made the choice to stop drinking, I hadn't threatened to leave or given him an ultimatum. He simply knew it was time to put the pieces of his life back together and learn to live with the tragic loss of his father. Since then, we've moved beyond those troubles, and I can only pray that since his renewed devotion to our marriage and to himself, he won't seek solace there again.

He called me from the car phone on their way there. He was crying and telling me how difficult it was for him to be away from me. It seems that when I am strong, he is weak, and the reverse remains true.

When he got to our house on Tuesday night, he called.

"I walk through this house and everything I see reminds me of you. I can smell you and see you in everything around me. I know I can't be away from you for two weeks. I can hardly stand to sleep in our bed without you," he cried.

As difficult as the distance between us has been on me, it seems that the hours of my days pass quickly and slowly at the same time. I believe God continues to rescue me from moments that are too painful to bear. It's the only mechanism I have discovered thus far, and if it appears to be denial, then I embrace it, escaping from a moment of utter fear and saving myself from the taunting of my uncertain fate. I sprint to my place of solitude and find myself somewhere between the day it came and waking to this morning.

When Wesley first told his brother, Wayne, that I had cancer, Wayne said he wanted to postpone his wedding until I got well and could be there to participate in it. I have known Wayne as long as I have known Wesley and our closeness over the years formed a bond that truly surpassed the fact that we ended up becoming family.

He and his fiancée, Tara, were already planning their wedding for March 30, so we convinced him to go on with their original plans and not wait on me. I don't expect them to postpone their wedding for me. Who knows what will become of this life by then. I can barely manage to cope with today.

I am scheduled for my first chemotherapy treatment tomorrow morning at 9:00 A.M., and my parents and Beverly are going with me. It is hard to believe that tomorrow is the day I start the medicine that will make me bald and recognizably sick to all. I ask myself again, "How did I get here?"

My dad will be leaving to work in Oregon this weekend, so my mom will be left to care for me on her own. I think she is frightened, but my dad has been working along the West Coast since I was in fifth grade. She has traveled with him since my brother and I left home after high school. They had even planned to leave together after the holidays and lease their house here, but that all changed when we found out about the cancer.

As strong as my dad tries to appear, I don't think he can handle watching what might come with chemotherapy. My mother is instinctively stronger than he is. She's nursed her babies back to health before. Must this be any different?

Dr. Verma's nurse, Kim, tried to prepare me for tomorrow. The hospital is walking distance from their office and has a separate entrance for chemotherapy patients, so patients can avoid areas of the hospital where sick people are being treated since our immune systems are compromised by the very drugs that are supposed to make us well. I guess it will get worse long before it gets better.

Friday, January 13

10:45 A.M.—I went to chemotherapy this morning. Or should I say, I attempted chemotherapy this morning.

The nurse gave my parents and me blue note cards that had the name of each drug I would be taking written down with the common side effects each causes. On the back of the cards were the side effects that were less common and more serious. If any of these occurred, I was supposed to call my doctor immediately. I opted not to read the back of the blue cards, because I knew if I read about the serious possibilities, my mind would play tricks on me and one or many of them would appear to pose a threat to my well-being. I needed to keep what was left of my peace of mind where these drugs were concerned, so I gave them to my mom and will let her and Wesley (who will be returning for all my other treatments) know if I experience anything other than what is considered common as treatments progressed.

My dad listened as the nurse spoke to us, but every time she left the room to get something, he buried his head in a magazine, as if what he was pretending to read could alleviate the tension of watching it all transpire. My father is not a weak man, but he is just a man.

My mom sat next to me and held my hand, telling me everything would be okay. I was right, my mom was better able to cope with the reality of watching her daughter start chemotherapy. My dad, however, was unable to participate fully, rendering solace from a magazine. Since when did he read *Cosmopolitan*?

After the nurse explained the many side effects of my treatment regimen and gave me the business cards of people who specialize in providing wigs and fill-in makeup tips for patients who'd lost their hair, she took my temperature.

She put the digital thermometer in my mouth and both of us watched as the numbers crept up slowly. We waited for them to stop somewhere near 98.5 degrees. When it exceeded 100 degrees, the nurse and I looked at each other with concern. "Are you feeling warm today?" she asked.

"No, in fact, I feel like I am cold all of the time," I answered.

"Like you have the chills?"

"Yes, exactly."

The thermometer finally stopped at 100.5 degrees. "Lisa, this fever is too high. I can't start your therapy knowing your temperature is likely to further rise as much as two or more degrees from the chemo."

By then, my dad had put the magazine down and Bev was kneeling down in front of my mom, holding her hand.

"You can go over to Dr. Verma's office, and he'll tell you what we should do from here," the nurse explained.

"What does this mean?" my dad asked.

"It could be the cancer causing the fever, but Dr. Verma will want to make sure there isn't another cause. Don't worry. This is actually okay, because some people who have cancer are unable to produce a fever at all because their body is unable to fight infection. Just go talk to him. He may even send you back over today."

"How late will you be here?" I asked. It took too much strength to prepare for this day to have it delayed any further.

"I'll be here as long as you need. I'll call and let him know you are on your way. He'll know what to do," she said, trying to lend comfort to our confusion.

When we arrived at his office, he asked me to spit some of the mucus I was coughing into a clear, plastic cup—the same kind the other doctor put my bone marrow in. I told him I wasn't good at coughing up phlegm, but he left me in his office to try.

After a few minutes of unsuccessful attempts, I asked my dad to come in the office to show me how. It was comical— my dad was trying to teach his daughter how to spit so the lab could test the results and see what else could be wrong as if cancer wasn't enough to deal with.

When I failed to produce a sample after attempting for more than ten minutes, Dr. Verma sent me home with the plastic cup and asked me to provide a sample to the lab by

1:00 P.M. so they could test it and have the results by 4:00 P.M. He gave me a prescription for an antibiotic to have filled in case it was simply an infection from the cough I had.

I took the cup home and finally gave up trying at 12:50 P.M. and called Dr. Verma's office. I jokingly asked my parents, "Can't I just blow my nose and give him that? They might not know the difference." They laughed long and hard about that. It was good to see them smile.

Coughing up phlegm was one of those things I could only do by accident, so Dr. Verma finally gave up and told me to take the antibiotics and if the fever was not down by Monday, then we could assume it was from the cancer and not a secondary infection. I'm scheduled to see him Monday afternoon.

There were flowers waiting for me when I got home from Wesley's mom and her husband, Roger. They, like us, thought I would be starting treatment today.

It's frustrating to not begin treatment, because I know that I am simply delaying the inevitable. I guess it will all catch up to me and soon enough I will embark upon the measures we must take in attempts to rid my young body of cancer. With each day I am forced to wait, I try hard not to imagine the cancer growing inside of me. Instead, I try to believe that this, too, shall pass.

Six

Monday, January 16

10:45 P.M.—For the past two hours, I have been trying to recover from a phone call I received from a woman who had breast cancer a year and a half ago. She heard about me from my friend, Jamie, and called to discuss my treatment choices. I didn't ask her to call me, and I was quite overwhelmed by the horrific things she had to say about the treatment regimen that she knew I had already chosen.

Among many other negative things she said about conventional treatment, she told me that her sister had cancer years before and chemotherapy had killed her. I could not believe my ears. She said that she herself refused to have chemotherapy and went on to rid herself of cancer with herbs and other alternative methods. Although I agreed with the many things she had to say about the importance of good nutrition and a positive attitude, I did not agree with her fear tactics.

What upset me the most were her unsolicited opinions of my choices for treatment. She tried to offer comfort when she began to sense my panic by saying that what mattered most was a belief in what I was choosing and its ability to help me in the healing process, but it was too late for comfort from her. In a short conversation, she managed to deplete what strength I mustered toward my choice of battle and send me into an orbit of doubt and confusion.

When we hung up the phone, I cried to my mother and confessed my fears to her. She was furious with that woman for managing to further batter me in my brittle state. She told me to call my brother and get in touch with Heather's aunt who had conquered Hodgkin's disease eighteen years ago.

Within five minutes of calling Vance, I was talking to Gina and was feeling a sense of peace from the moment she spoke. She, too, believed in the holistic measures a person could take in the healing process, but she also believed in conventional therapies for treatment. Gina had stage IV Hodgkin's at a time when many doctors were still trying to figure out the best way to treat it. I took comfort in her words and in her philosophy that you must take responsibility for your own health and utilize every possible avenue for recovery. You must believe first in your ability to survive with the help of family, doctors and faith, and leaving one of those components out entirely could hinder your ability to battle.

Vance and Heather gave me the greatest hope by sending me Gina. She has literally entered my life as a ray of hope—a tenderness and peace that, in just a few weeks, I had begun to believe would not exist for me. She brought me out of orbit and for that I am thankful, because there is nothing like the voice of a survivor.

I later called Jamie and told her that I didn't want her friend to call me again. I was angry about the woman's choice of words and her tactics and that kind of advice was not welcome in my home. At first, Jamie was defensive, because I know she was only trying to help, but I explained to her that she might not be able to fully understand or participate in what my family was going through. What made me most angry with that woman for calling me the night before beginning treatment was the fact that she never bothered to tell me that she was dealing with a possible recurrence. She led me to believe that she had cured herself of cancer, and it was only after speaking with Jamie that I learned the truth.

I don't think it's a good idea to confuse the issues of treatment further by the advice of others who do not agree with my choices. I am also returning my mom's friend Carlita's nursing book. I know that some people would find it helpful, but it holds too much information for me to handle right now. There is something to be said for an informed decision, but I am learning that it is within one's own reasoning.

Despite this setback, I am ready for chemotherapy tomorrow. Or should I say, ready as I will ever be? I went to my appointment this afternoon and discovered I still have a fever. Dr. Verma said it is presumably from the cancer itself and has arranged for me to start chemotherapy tomorrow morning. He said it would be better to start earlier in the week rather than just before the weekend, in case I have any complications or need to visit his office in the early days after starting the therapy.

My parents and I celebrated my dad's forty-seventh birthday a day early with a sour cream lemon pie last night. He left for Oregon this morning. It's just my mom and me now. Set to battle . . .

Tuesday, January 17

5:53 A.M.—Just before the sunlight shines through my window this morning, I watch the street lights dim and see the paper boy delivering the morning news, and I know that today is the first day of what has come to find me—what has come to find the others. I watch the birds come alive in the trees and listen to their song, imagining they are singing just for me.

Through my bedroom window, I see the comings of the day—and through this window, I see what is expected of me, what I must do. Unlike the days before and the days to come, this is one like no other. It's the day I choose for myself what is to be my life's battle. The fight, the struggle, the serenity I have always heard of, finds me here, standing in front of my window, and I am asked to choose what it will be for myself.

The morning moments are quiet and while I imagine him sleeping in our bed, even though he is still far away, I see him take each breath with ease and understand that although this task is easy for him, so many other things in his life are not. I wonder why it took us so long to find each other and now face this choice, this reasoning of my heart. And as he sleeps, I pray quietly to myself my prayer of thanks for all that came to my life before him and for all that has come to my life since him.

The morning remains quiet, and I try to be silent for my mother to spare her the early morning realization that comes when something inside is broken, something that I never even knew I had, and something I continue to pray is not lost forever.

My time here is amongst the most rewarding gifts a person could know. I haven't traveled the world or accomplished scholarly triumphs, but I have lived and I have loved. I have triumphed in the knowledge that the people in my life are the only people with whom I would ever choose to share my life. The word "choose" comes to my mind again, and I begin to understand in the wee morning hours of this day that what I have awakened for is the gift of my life. In the quiet moments of this stillness, I begin to see the journey ahead of me, and I begin to trust that whatever is to come is what I shall fight for. And just as the others fight for me, I, too, fight for myself. I fight for my life.

I may never travel the world, but I have traveled to the place that finds me here—the place that gives me enough love to understand and reckon with the uncertainty. And so, with the gifts of my life, I choose to fight, I choose to live, and I choose to begin on this day to do whatever it takes to be here for another day.

And as the quiet morning leaves and the house awakens, I imagine that I see him open his eyes and watch me stand next to my window. He doesn't speak. He just smiles, and as his eyes begin to shine, I can feel the light inside me begin again, and I know that I am home. And for as long as I live, this is the place I will always be with him—home.

There are few things to be certain of in life. But I believe in the certainty of hope, and I believe in God's love for me and for those before and after me. And I know that with each day I begin, I will come to understand the significance of my journey. And as I awaken to the song of the same birds again tomorrow and stand again in front of my window with Wesley one day closer to returning, I know that with all that is good in the world, I will be healed. And this alone gives me the strength to face tomorrow with the love that shines in the eyes of Wesley. . . . For all things can be seen through the love that shines in the eyes of Wesley.

5:14 P.M.— Bev and Jeri, my dad's brother's wife, left a little while ago. When we first got home from chemotherapy we all seemed to be sitting and waiting for something to happen.

I arrived at the hospital with my mom at 9:00 A.M. sharp. Bev and Jeri met us there and were waiting by the entrance when we arrived. I have never known Bev to be on time, but today she was. There was a different nurse there then last time, but she seemed equally nice and her name was also Mary.

The chemotherapy room had reclining chairs for the patients and a few chairs for others to sit in. The room also had a TV and magazines. Mary thought we would be more comfortable in the waiting room for the patients' families, because there were so many of us. That room was comfortable and also had a recliner for me to sit in, along with two love seats for the others and a TV. I don't think patients usually brought such an entourage with them to treatment, but I brought them because I needed their support. I made no excuses for it, and Mary accommodated us nicely.

We were able to skip all of the note cards this time and got started right away. The large needle hurt going into my hand, and when my mom saw my pain she had to get up and leave the room. She didn't want me to see her cry. She soon returned and seemed to be as ready as the rest of us to begin.

After the needle was in, Mary taped it tightly to my hand, then taped my hand to a board that forced my hand to stay in place, wrapping my fingers around the board's edge. She said it would insure that the needle stayed in place to prevent tissue damage once the chemotherapy was administered through the IV.

Mary started each drug by telling me what it was called and what initial reactions my body might have to it. Just about every drug I received that was part of the ABVD regimen had another drug to go along with it to prevent an adverse reaction. Mary started with Benadryl, and, as soon as it hit my vein, I started seeing double. I have never taken drugs, so Benadryl by mouth, let alone by IV, made me high. I didn't like the feeling it gave me—like I was somewhat out of control of things, but that wasn't the worst of it.

One of the nausea medications I received near the beginning of treatment was called Decadron. Mary warned me that I would experience some itching around my buttocks, but that was an understatement. As soon as the drug hit the

IV, I felt this horrible itching sensation that started at the tip of my head and worked its way down to my feet. In between, it remained in my crotch area for at least two minutes. It was the worst itching I had ever felt—even worse than the way the cancer made me itch. It was like all of the months I had suffered with itching were concentrated in one area of my body. And since it was in such a place that scratching hardly seemed appropriate, I suffered through it.

I can't remember the name or initial side effect of every drug she gave me, but there were a few that I won't soon forget. She had to give me a test dose of Bleomycin, because it can cause some people to have an increased heart rate, among other things. It made me nervous to receive the test dose, but she reassured me that giving me only one milligram of the drug would be enough for them to know how I would react to the entire dose. Everything went fine, so she gave me the full dose.

Velban was the worst drug, because it hurt so badly going in. It felt like pure rubbing alcohol going into my veins, and the only relief I got from the pain was to have my forearm rubbed the entire time the drug was being administered through the IV drip. My mom and the others took turns rubbing my arm and literally had to rub it constantly. If they stopped, the pain was too much to bear. The drug took a long time to administer, because it was difficult to find a place for it to enter that I could tolerate. A few times I asked her to speed it up just so I could get it over with, but she would immediately have to slow it down again, because the pain was so great. Mary said that my tiny veins were probably what caused such discomfort. I hadn't expected to feel pain during chemotherapy, so I was very upset by what was happening.

Partway through treatment, I started to listen to my headphones and the CD I had brought with me when I started to cry. All the words made me sad, and suddenly I realized where I was and what was happening to me. A rush of emotions ran through me. Mostly I just felt a bitter sadness for what was taking place and, above all, I wondered how in the world I had gotten there. Bev saw me crying and removed my headphones.

"Why are you crying?" she asked.

"The music must have hit me. I haven't been listening to music at all since this started, not even in the car," I answered.

"You just leave the headphones off and stay here with us," she said. So I did.

"Would you like to have something to help take the edge off?" Mary asked.

"What do you mean?" I asked.

"There's a drug called Ativan that I could give you that would still enable you to know what is going on, but you just won't care as much," she answered, knowing that I preferred not to have drugs that made me feel out of control of my body.

I didn't answer her; I just looked puzzled about what to do.

"I can call Dr. Verma to see if he'll let you have it, then you can decide," she suggested. I agreed.

Mary ordered lunch for us at about 11:00 A.M. I ordered a turkey sandwich and grapes. I was surprised that I actually felt like I could eat.

After she ordered lunch, she came back in with a new needle that had Ativan in it.

Dr. Verma had given the okay for it. I thought I wanted it, but when she put it up to the IV and was started to administer it, I changed my mind.

"No, stop. I don't want it," I told her. No questions asked—she stopped and laid it on the shelf near my cranberry-grape juice and my Sprite.

"Okay, but it's here if you change your mind."

The whole treatment ended up taking about seven hours. It seemed like longer. Throughout the treatment, Mary checked my IV and made sure that it had "good flow" and wasn't irritating my hand. I had to have help going to the bathroom, because I could only use one hand. My mom pushed my IV cart and held on to me while we walked to the bathroom. I had a hard time keeping my balance at different times, because of the Benadryl and other drugs, but my mom held me tightly. I also experienced severe chills during parts of treatment. Mary said that was common and gave me some blankets.

When it was all over, Mary gave me some Compazine and Tylenol to take home. She said to take the Tylenol every four hours for the next two days to prevent fever and the Compazine every four hours for the rest of the day and whenever needed after that. The Compazine was to prevent nausea, so she said it was most helpful to take it at the first onset of nausea. She also gave me a journal to note my side effects in and told me to look for patterns, so I would know when to take the nausea medication before the nausea actually caused me any discomfort.

Mary has been an oncology nurse for more than twenty years, so she knows the tricks of her trade and shared them openly. Even though she had never experienced the adverse events that accompanied chemotherapy, she was good at explaining them in a way that helped prepare me for what was coming. I liked her immensely and was glad to have such a caring nurse. I trusted her and felt blessed once again to have another competent health care professional taking care of me. I couldn't imagine going through it any other way.

Now that it's over and I have a better understanding of the process, chemotherapy isn't much like they make it seem in the movies. For many others and me, all we can anticipate going into this is what we have seen in the media. I kept thinking that I would be violently ill, but so far I feel pretty good. It's a difficult thing to bear, no matter how it's perceived. The possibilities alone make me scared of what might come when the drugs begin to do their work, but I also have a better understanding of what would come without these drugs, and I am not ready to give up and die. This fight has only just begun.

People speak about the fight and wonder how I can be so strong. I think this strength is in each of us, but sometimes one person is tested more than another is. Overall, we are as strong as we choose to be and, for now, I am managing to be as strong as my family helps me to be. If I had to be separated from everyone but Wesley and was expected to go through this with only him, I could do it. But fortunately, God brought me here for the holidays and Wesley and I do not have to go through it without the support of my family.

The waiting room where I received treatment is a place where I never thought I would be. This whole experience is a place I never thought I would be. But rather than question why or how, I guess it's time to just focus on the business at hand. The drugs hurt, and they weaken my body and my spirit, but I am willing to allow them to become my friend and my enemy. It's a choice. It's the best I can do today.

Thursday, January 19

8:10 P.M.—Each day I wondered what would happen to my body once the drugs began to work, and today it came. The suffering began.

I still haven't been eating very much, so when I woke up this morning I felt weak in my knees. I started the morning in the bathroom with severe diarrhea and shakes. I could barely hold myself up on the toilet. When I began to sweat, I tried to finish in the bathroom and go back to bed. On my way, I yelled to my mom in the kitchen and asked her to bring me a nausea pill. The rest is a blur.

The next thing I remember is waking up on the cold floor, rooting my head and my knees into the tile. When I realized where I was, I quickly got up and got into bed. It all must have happened fast, because when my mom entered the room with my pill, I asked her what took so long. She said it had only been a couple minutes. My head and knees were skinned from the fall and my body was still shaking.

"It's here, Mom. This is it. This is bad," I said to her in a panic.

"You just haven't been getting enough to eat. I'll go get you some bananas," she said as she left the room. I sensed her panic as well.

She returned with the bananas. "From now on, you take a nausea pill before you get out of bed and call for me to bring you something to eat on the days you feel sick. You have to be careful."

The pamphlets had warned against getting any injuries or infections, because it could delay treatment with a compromised immune system. If the doctor preferred that I not even shave my legs with a regular razor because it could cut me and cause infection, then I figured a knot on the head was a really bad idea.

As my mom stood there feeding me bananas, I felt very scared and alone. Despite her help, I felt like the worst had arrived, and I felt lonely in my misery. Everyone is struggling in his or her own way with what is happening to me, but I still felt that as much as they all try to understand, I am the one waking up with my face digging into the floor and not knowing why.

When I got up from bed, I called Bev and asked her to come over and help us through the day.

"Can you come over today?" I asked her.

"Yes," she answered without question.

"It's starting," I told her.

"I'll be there in an hour."

She and my cousin, Darla, spent the day with us. Having them here was helpful. It took my mind off of how badly I was feeling. Together, we watched as the pure white snow fell outside for the first time in years. It fell at a time when my day could stand to be brightened by something pure. I took pictures from the window of Huck playing in the snow and even though I couldn't go outside and risk catching a cold, it made me happy to just watch from the window.

I spent most of the day in and out of the bathroom. The nausea pills took the edge off but hardly relieved my discomfort completely. At the end of the day, I feel tired and ragged from the toll the treatment is beginning to take. I hope tomorrow will be better.

Friday, January 19

3:14 A.M.—It's the middle of the night. Wesley called me before he went to bed. He misses me. I know he thought that going back to Texas was the right thing to do and that gathering our things to bring back with him for the duration of our stay would give him a chance to regroup for what is ahead. But now that he is there, I think he wishes he were still here with me. There is nothing that we can to say to each other about our plight. We are both trying to be strong. Some days are easier than others are, but every single day is a struggle. I long for his return and for his presence here with me. Since the day we came together, his everyday presence in my life has sustained me through many things. And it is with his love and his help that I expect to gather enough strength to continue this fight. I turn to God and to my family, but lately, it seems that nothing gets me through a moment more than the voice of that man telling me I will survive. Whether or not he truly believes it, I do not yet know, but as long as he keeps saying it when I ask, I think I will get through many uncertain moments.

I have been going through old family photo albums. I hadn't looked through them in a long time. I always loved looking at them, but now when I see a picture of me as a baby or as a small child, I say to myself, "In twenty-four years you are going to get cancer." I try not to let it take away from the precious memories the photos represent, but I find it very difficult not to realize that everything I ever did in my life has brought me here. When I look at the pictures of different times in all of our lives, I realize I didn't know then that those events made up my childhood and my life. It's only after those years have passed that I can fully appreciate them for their true importance. Unlike before this happened to me, I don't wish I could go back to change any point in my life preceding December 26, because all roads would lead me right back to here. Once I leave here, I'll go forward forever.

I just took another bath to try and relieve the itching. I trust what Mary said about the itching going away once the chemo begins to work. What will it be like to have a whole night's sleep without this misery and discomfort? It seems like it's been months since I have had any relief from the constant and relentless mutation of the insides of my body. What could have possibly been going on inside of me to make everything go so wrong? It's still a mystery to me.

My mom is asleep on the other end of the couch. Neither of us made it to bed tonight. I don't want to wake her. We've had a hard night. I started to get a fever again at about 7:00 P.M. My mom and I had to take my temperature every hour for several hours. While we watched movies on television, we charted my temperature and crossed our fingers that it would remain below 101 degrees. I just kept hearing Dr.

Verma's words, "As long as your fever remains below 101, you can take Tylenol to control it, and you won't have to be hospitalized."

I was so scared last night. I could see that my mom was worried as well. With both my dad and Wesley out of town, she had to remain strong while caring for me. There was hurt in her eyes when I began to cry.

"I hate this, Mom. I hate all of it. This fever is scaring me," I said as tears streamed down my face.

"I hate it too, Lisa. But you are fine. Your fever is staying under 101. You'll be fine," my mom reassured me.

"But what if I go to sleep and my fever goes over 101, and I don't know it?" I questioned her.

"You'll know if you have a higher fever. Do you remember when you were a little girl and you would get sick and come to our bedroom wanting to sleep with me and your dad?"

"Yeah, I remember."

"Well, you woke up because you were sick and your body was telling you that something was wrong. You'll be fine, Lisa. I'll set my clock for every four hours. We'll take your temperature, then you can take Tylenol to keep it down."

"I wish it were like that now. I wish that all I had to do to feel better was crawl into the warmth and safety of you and Dad."

"That's what we wish, too," my mom admitted.

"I'm so afraid, Mom. I'm so afraid of everything that is happening to me. I know that the chemo is going to make me well, but it's hurting my body while it does. It just keeps showing itself to me differently throughout each day. I don't know how sick I will get before it stops. I don't even know if it's working," I confided. I had been lying with my legs in her lap, and she was scratching them while we talked. She did it to help relieve the itching.

"I know, Lisa. But you've got to believe that you are going to get through this. You have to help your body get well."

I turned around to lay my head in her lap. She ran her fingers through my hair while I continued confessing my fears. "Mom, you seem so sad. Are you sad because you are afraid I might die, or are you sad because of all I have to go through to get better?"

"I know you are going to be all right. I really believe that. I am just sad for all you have to go through to get there."

"Are you afraid, Mom?"

"No, I know you will survive. I just hate to watch you suffering. Are you always afraid, Lisa?" my mom asked.

"All of the time, Mom. Every minute. From the moment I wake up until the moment I go to sleep it is with me. I am afraid. Sometimes when I wake up in the morning, for just a split-second I forget, but then I open my eyes and I remember. I'm lying in my old bedroom with Wesley, and I remember why I am here. And no matter what else I think about being in my childhood room, I know I am only here because I am so sick. And with all of my heart I pray I have not returned home to die. I am always afraid."

"Is there ever a moment when you are not afraid? Is there ever a moment when you feel free of this?" my mom further questioned, trying to help me find a moment's peace.

"Yes."

"When is it, Lisa? When are you not afraid?"

Through the tears, I managed a reply, "Only when I sleep."

As she placed her hands over my warm face, she wiped away the tears that were still flowing slowly down my trembling cheeks. My mom spoke softly, "Then sleep, Lisa." I closed my eyes as she wiped my tears. "Just go to sleep."

So I did. And for several hours, I rested. And for several hours, while I slept in the lap and the safety of my mother's love, my body fought to heal, and I was not afraid.

Seven

Tuesday, January 22

Wesley is on his way back from Texas. We have spoken every day that he has been gone, and he is eager to get back to me. He plans to stop in Sacramento to see our friends, John and Kirsten, because he will arrive in Sacramento very late on Thursday night, so I thought I might drive there and surprise him. My mom doesn't think it's a good idea.

I have been feeling pretty good all week. The weekend was rough, but once I figured out that some days the most I am able to do is get dressed and rest on the couch, I am coping better with my limitations. Friends have been coming to visit and "get well" cards have started to come in the mail daily from people wanting to lend their support. My dad calls every day, sometimes several times a day, to check on us. Vance also continues to call and wants to come home to see me as soon as possible. He doesn't know when he will be able to. Mostly, I just want Wesley to get back. To say that I have missed him barely lends a glimpse into the emptiness I have felt since he left, although my mother has been wonderful and is taking good care of me.

My appetite is starting to return and, best of all, the itching has slightly diminished. It is still quite bad, but it is getting better with treatment just like Mary said it would. I spent the night at my Aunt Jeri and Uncle Tommy's one night last week. My grandma has lived with them and their two children, Ryan and Krystal, since my grandpa died. It was good to spend time with them.

Jeri made me a grilled cheese sandwich that took me all day to eat. I was itching badly during the night, so she gave me Ryan's bedspread to use. It's much more comfortable than the one that's on my bed now. Ryan's is cotton and doesn't have any lace or feathers. She let me take it home until the itching subsides completely.

My dad wants my mom to go up to Washington and visit him for a week, but she is apprehensive about leaving me. I know I will be fine once Wesley gets back, but my dad has not been able to talk her into going. Maybe she'll change her mind when Wesley returns. It must be difficult for my dad to be alone. When he called to see how I was feeling last weekend, he had a hard time listening to my answer. I think he asked the question because he should but wanted me to tell him it wasn't so bad. It hurt him to know I was suffering but not nearly as much as the suffering itself.

For the next few days, I will wait for Wesley and be here for his calls along the way. I am scheduled for my second treatment on January 30, so Wesley will be here in time for it. I think he is dreading the process but wants to be here to help me through.

Thursday, January 25

12:14 A.M.—I felt like a teenager waiting on my date for the prom in the hours before Wesley arrived. He called and said he wouldn't be stopping in Sacramento to sleep. He was too close to me to stop.

I met him at the door when he arrived and hugged him for as long as I could stand the cold outside. He looked new to me, like a breath of fresh air, and I knew that having him with me again would help get me through this. My mom left us to our privacy while Wesley and I talked at the kitchen table about all that we had missed in the days he'd been gone.

We soon went to bed. Having him next to me felt like nothing had in the days that he was gone. It gave me a sense of peace and comfort knowing he was there, and his strong arms gave me a place of retreat. Tears began to fall from my eyes but soon disappeared with each touch and whisper of his love. He was home again and for the first time since the bad news had come, we made our way to love.

Monday, January 29

Kim, Dr. Verma's nurse, called and asked me to go to the lab before going to the office for my afternoon appointment. She said it was standard procedure to have my blood work done before going forward with the next treatment.

I was the youngest person at the lab. There was a woman there who had been going through numerous tests because she has a blood disease that doctors were having a difficult time diagnosing and treating. I guess things could be worse for me. At least I know what I have and the doctors seem confident about how to treat it. It was a comfort at first, but I think I will scream if I hear one more health care professional tell me that I have the best kind of cancer to get. Such a thing does not exist.

Bev was here today when I received the news that I wouldn't be having my second chemotherapy tomorrow as scheduled. I was very upset and confused, especially since I knew it was very important to stay on schedule with the protocol for treatment, giving me the best chance of kicking the cancer while it was down and having a full recovery. Kim explained that my white blood cell count, the blood cells that fight infection, was only 2.4 and it needed to be at least 5.0 in order for me to go through another treatment. I didn't know what to say to her when she told me, so I just said goodbye and hung up the phone confused and disappointed.

"What's the matter?" my mom asked.

"That was Kim. She said I couldn't have treatment tomorrow, because I do not have enough white blood cells left."

"What does that mean?" Bev asked.

"I have absolutely no idea. She said that I have to have enough to fight infection and if I have another treatment right now, then I will be left with too few or even none at all."

"So what did she say they are going to do?" my mom asked, looking as confused as I was.

"They don't do anything. She said we just have to wait another week and see if it comes back up. I don't understand what any of this means."

"Well, did you ask her any more questions while you had her on the phone?" my mom pressed further.

"I was in shock. I didn't know what to ask. I just said okay and hung up the phone."

"Do you want me to call her back and have her explain it again?" Bev asked.

"Would you?"

"Sure, hon."

Bev left the room to call the nurse back, while I sat and waited for her to return with new information that could somehow shed some light on the situation. The phone call was brief, but Bev came back into the room with some answers. Not the answers I wanted to hear, but some answers at least.

"Okay. This is how it works," Bev began. "Right now your

white blood cell count is 2.4, which means your immune system is extremely compromised. When the chemo fights the bad cells in your body it also fights the good, so your body has to work harder to keep up. If you had treatment now, you would be left without any white blood cells at all until your body could produce more. In the meantime, you could get very sick from something as simple as a common cold, which would delay your treatment more than just waiting for your white blood cells to return to normal."

"So my white blood cells will return?" I questioned.

"Oh yeah. Your body is constantly making blood cells, and it's routine for the doctor to have you wait an extra week for the cells to catch up before continuing."

"So this has happened before. It's kind of routine?" I asked.

"Yes. Just wait out another week, and you will go back for treatment."

It was beginning to make sense to me, but I just felt that things were getting so much more complicated with each day that passed. Sometimes I felt like I had a handle on things, and other times I felt like the whole ordeal was spinning out of control.

5:46 P.M.—When Wesley got home from grocery shopping, I explained to him that I wouldn't be having another treatment until the following Tuesday. He didn't seem upset or concerned by it. He figured that Dr. Verma knew what he was doing and it was better to be safe than sorry.

I explained the same to my dad when he called me from Oregon that night. I could tell when he called that he wanted to talk about something more than how I was feeling.

"Well, your mom was going to wait until later in the week to talk with you about this. But since there has been a delay, maybe we should talk about it now," my dad began.

"Talk to me about what?" I asked.

"Well. . . you understand that you come first right now. Whatever you need, whatever is going to get you through this the best possible way is what your mom and I want for you. You know that right?"

"Yeah. Why are you saying all of this? What's the matter?" I asked, concerned about where this could be heading.

"I have been asking your mom to come and spend a week with me, but she is concerned about leaving you."

"She doesn't need to be," I replied.

"I know, but she just wants to stay and help Wesley with your next treatment before leaving. She wants to be able to help him while you are sick. She also doesn't want to miss your treatment."

"Dad, I understand she is reluctant to leave because she will miss the actual treatment process, but she doesn't need to stay for that. She certainly doesn't need to stay to help Wesley take care of me. He can handle it. If you want her with you and she wants to go, then she shouldn't feel guilty about that. We'll be fine."

"You come first. If you want her there, then I will still come this weekend, and then go back by myself."

"Dad, tell her it's fine. Or I'll tell her."

"Okay, hon. If you're sure."

"That's enough. I'm sure. As long as I have Wesley here, I'll be fine."

I know that as much as my dad wants to be here for my treatments and to support my mother, he's always had to travel for his job. He's worked on dams in Oregon and Washington repairing hydroelectric generators since I was ten years old, so we have almost grown used to him being gone a lot of the time. He had to go where there was work and has now created a lucrative career for himself.

Since I left home, my mom has traveled with him during

the months of the year that required him to be gone, but she has stayed behind this time to help take care of me. When I was a child, he traveled so my parents could better support our family, and now that I am an adult, his reasons for going are not any different. It's because of our family's support that Wesley and I are able to be here while I go through treatment. And as hard as it is for us all, particularly my mother, my dad will continue his schedule of only returning every other weekend to see us.

After my dad visits this weekend, my mom will go back with him for the week. I am looking forward to some time alone with Wesley and worrying less about what a nuisance Huck has been.

Huck has been getting into trouble and is being compared to the other dogs. Even though it's best that we are here going through this, it doesn't make it easy to deal with the same dynamics of my family that have always existed. Huck's shortcomings seem to be secondary. He's been chewing up whatever is laying around and not "going potty" in designated areas of the yard, but what makes it harder is the way my parents talk to me where he is concerned. While Vance's dog, Gazlen, is here and receiving the best of care because she is older and well-behaved, Huck is getting put in the garage rather than in my room where he sleeps when he has a good day.

It seems that when I enter the doors of this house, all of the old rules still apply. It's never been a question of love or my parent's commitment to my brother and me; it's just this subtlety that has followed us in the differences of how we were raised. I grew up having different rules than Vance. My parents weren't strict, but what was required of me, such as an earlier curfew and no one of the opposite sex being allowed in my bedroom, was not required of my brother.

Vance would say that my hang-ups are just that, hang-ups

about what has or has not been fair to me because of the differences between how a boy and how a girl can be raised in a house where some of the old rules still apply. I guess that's because none of my hang-ups have directly affected his life. He was very good at leaving and moving on to a life separate from here. I think that's just what sons do, while daughters tend to linger and continue to seek approval from the parents who coddled them throughout their lives.

None of this is any different from what a lot of people tell me they have experienced in their own families, but at a time like this, I just don't want to be told what to do. Wesley sometimes battles with it, because he sees the way they both treat me like a child and how I respond. Before him, I used to allow much of their coaxing to determine many of my decisions in life. I guess that came more from my own eagerness to please and not disappoint them. Since Wesley and I have been together, I have become more independent of them but have also lived two thousand miles away from this house and the child I was when I lived in it.

In all of this, Vance's absence has been difficult. I am used to his absence, but I think my parents would feel better having him here through some of it. But because it's winter, Vance must ski the highest mountains and hope that the photos make it to print. It's what he does. I understand that.

Vance and Heather will be here in April, and truly all I want to do is hold him then. All of these other things that seem to matter less and less as this experience wears on will just fall away. I have felt for many years now that the time Vance and I spend together has been better spent than it was during the years we were growing up. We hated each other then, and I think we both had to realize our differences didn't make either one of us better than the other, just different— my city, his mountains.

I know these things will work themselves out. When I first

found out I was sick, I asked my dad if he was sure they could handle us being here for an indefinite period of time. He assured me they could. Having two married couples living under one roof is never easy, but I like to think that, given the circumstances, we can rise above our need to be heard. I like to think that's possible.

Friday, January 2

My dad arrived about an hour ago. It's good to have him home. My mom greeted him at the door and when the two hugged, they seemed to melt in each other's arms and remained still in that comfort until each of them released enough of what had been haunting them over the past several days. It was good to see them together, realizing this family has encountered other hardships, although none as horrible as this, but the one thing that has always managed to remain the same is that my parents love each other.

Tomorrow they will celebrate their thirtieth wedding anniversary. When I was a child and people saw my mom and dad together, they would ask me if he was my stepdad, because he had blond hair and blue eyes and my brother and I both looked so much like my mother. I used to ask, "What's a stepdad?" I truly didn't know. I was a lucky kid.

We do not have much planned for the weekend. Wesley wanted to go fishing, but it hasn't stopped raining for days and the river is up too high for fishing. We have very little money, so our choices for entertainment are limited. I am not supposed to go places where there are a lot of people, like movie theaters or shopping malls, because my immune system is compromised, so I can't be exposed to the season's colds and flu. Things can get rather boring, especially on the days when I feel good enough to venture beyond this house.

The itching has continued to diminish with each passing

day and, so far, I still have all of my hair. I am resigned to losing it. I figure that's better than being disappointed if it does fall out. My Grandma Shaw offered to buy me a wig if it does. Amber and I went looking yesterday, but all I found were wigs that didn't fit my personality. The saleswoman was trying to sell me something that she said would prevent my hair from falling out and had worked for other women. Mary already told me to stay clear of those products, because they had nothing to do with determining whether or not I would lose my hair. I believe her.

Monday, February 5

My mom and dad left early this morning. I could tell my mom was torn about going, but I reassured her that the time alone with our husbands would do us both some good. My dad seemed pleased to see that I was feeling well. I guess he got to be spared the reality of what those drugs do to my body, since I hadn't had treatment in three weeks.

I went for my blood work this morning. Kim called a little while ago to say I would be having treatment tomorrow. What a relief! My white blood cell count is back up to 8.3. When I talked to Laverne earlier today, I told her I would be having chemotherapy tomorrow and she said, "Oh, I am sorry to hear that."

I said, "Sorry! Don't be sorry. I have to have it to get well, so not having it only prolongs my illness. Having it is the most important thing."

She seemed shocked by my reply, but that doesn't surprise me. Laverne hasn't been around enough to comprehend what any of this means. I have called and asked her to invite my mom to a movie or to have a cup of coffee sometime. She said she would, but she never did. I don't expect everyone to deal with this in the same way, especially her because she's still coping with Alton's death, but she is my mom's friend. I don't understand why some people can't just admit their limitations when dealing with cancer.

Chemo is tomorrow. Mary says it gets easier each time. One can hope.

Tuesday, February 6

5:14 P.M.—We all used the waiting room again for treatment. Wesley, Bev, Jeri and Darla went with me this time. My mom not being there was probably harder on her than it was on me. I had Wesley.

The immediate effects of the drugs remained the same as the first time. Wesley rubbed my arm through most of the painful drug. Having him there made an enormous difference. He held my hand when she started my IV, and I cried. He helped me walk to the bathroom. He even laughed out loud when the anti-nausea medication that made my privates itch began to work. I squirmed in my seat a lot during that one. He did everything I needed him to do, but most of all he sat next to me and gave me a smile when I needed it. There's nothing like Wesley in a room with me when I feel some hope is lost. His love alone makes me want to survive.

Thursday, February 8

3:14 P.M.—As the chemo flows through my veins, I feel a sense of peace knowing that something is being done. I am feeling the same affects as last time, even a little less.

I am okay with my mom being gone. I know it's just geography, because I feel her every moment of every day. It's something between a mother and daughter. It's something I have learned even more about in the past weeks.

Now that I've had my second treatment, I realize that not having treatment was more difficult mentally than having it was physically. I just want something going in to get the cancer out.

Wesley continues to be an incredible help. He asked me earlier today, "When do I start taking care of you?"

Within hours of him asking, the diarrhea began and so did the chills and sweating. In between trips to the bathroom, I laid on the couch in a fetal position. Wesley looked sad watching me suffer through it. Short of bringing my nausea pill, there really wasn't much he could do for me. He rubbed my back and scratched my legs the way he used to before the itching had begun to subside. Within a few hours, the severe nausea passed and we were able to play a few games of Scrabble. Playing board games is all we seem to do around here lately.

While we were playing a game, I ran my fingers through my hair as I have been doing to see if it was starting to fall out. When I pulled my fingers away, there were several hairs between my fingers. I was shocked. I looked at Wesley, who looked equally shocked.

"Here we go," I said to him as I let the hair fall to the floor.

"Are you okay?" he asked me as he reached for my hand.

"I'm fine. We knew this would happen."

"Are you sure?" he questioned further.

"I'm more than sure. Draw a letter."

Eight

Monday, February 19

8:20 A.M.—I haven't been writing as much because of the pain in my hand. We got the treatment down to four hours last time, but four days later, my hand started to ache from the Velban drug that hurts going in. It hurts worse and longer than the first time. It feels better when I am up and walking around, which makes it difficult to get any decent rest, especially at night. I started sleeping with a heating pad around my hand and forearm. It hasn't been helping.

I am otherwise pretty pleased with the way my body seems to be responding to the chemotherapy. Dr. Verma plans to do a chest X-ray before the next treatment to get an assessment of how well the cancer is responding. He says that this type of cancer is less likely to come back than other types as long as we do enough now.

The side effects seem to come like clockwork as compared to the first round—almost to the hour, definitely to the day. The worst is how sore my mouth gets and the awful tastes that come with the soreness. The chemo seems to secrete

97

through my tongue and into my mouth, then when I swallow I get a stomachache. That usually lasts a little more than two days. I rinse my mouth often with warm water and baking soda. That gives me almost instant relief, but it doesn't last long. My tongue is swollen and tender. Wesley says it looks like a cooked chicken breast. I read that toxins are released through my tongue, which is partly the cause for the mouth sores. That makes sense because of all of the toxins I have inside of me trying to get out.

The weight loss has slowed down. Before treatment, I lost two pounds every four to five days. After the first chemo, the nausea wore off, and I got my appetite back for a few days and managed to gain a few pounds. Then, the cycle repeated itself with the second round of chemo. Being able to eat more this time has helped my energy level.

Wesley is picking up my parents at the airport in Sacramento tomorrow. He plans to find a part-time job since my mom will be here to help. He couldn't leave me alone some of the days I was sick. So far, I have avoided being left alone since this all started, and I still haven't listened to music. Wesley tried to turn on the stereo the other day while we were home alone, but I asked him not to, so he didn't. He didn't understand why.

"I just can't bear to hear the words," I told him.

"What words?" he asked.

"Anything sad or anything happy. Any words at all," I answered.

I can't explain why I don't want to be left alone. I spend so much of my time surrounded by the people who love me most that I have grown used to feeling their literal presence. There have been many times since the day I found out when I have felt very alone, even in a crowded room, but to actually be alone would mean that I would have to be alone with these thoughts, these fears. They overwhelm me sometimes.

I might be watching something on television or having a conversation with someone when the anguish of my reality surfaces. I say to myself, "You have cancer." And the words sound as unreal to me as they did when Dr. McCabe said them to me weeks ago. Nothing seems to make it more real than it is, because I still can't figure out how I got here, why I got here. In these moments of realization, I sometimes wait for an epiphany from God—some light to shine brightly on me and lead me to understanding. But the epiphany eludes me, and I am left with the uncertainties I cannot manage to smother, and truly the only thing I know for sure is that I won't allow myself to imagine the demise this disease could bring. What mind could allow that to creep in?

11:15 A.M.—The weather has been beautiful. Everyone is walking around in shorts with white legs, except for those who frequent tanning beds. I have been to them off and on throughout my adult life, but I will never go to one again. Not ever! After being diagnosed, taking unnecessary risks that could lead to another form of cancer is unthinkable to me. I am not even allowed in the direct sunlight right now, at least for prolonged periods of time. It makes me nauseous.

There are a lot of limitations that have come with this type of treatment, but the worst is the social isolation. I can't be around sick people or recently immunized children. Jeri won't let her daughter, Krystal, get her shots for school, because she would have to stay away from me for a while. The school isn't happy about it, but Jeri told them I have cancer and she will not allow her family to be isolated from me.

Wesley got his ticket for Wayne's wedding. I talked to Wayne tonight about my not being able to go. He was sweet about it, telling me he understands and loves me. I don't want to fly and risk getting sick on the trip. I figure that as long as I keep my eye on the big picture and make these sacrifices that can help keep me on schedule with treatment, all of this will be worth it. Besides, my hair is falling out more and more each day, and I don't care to make my first appearance looking gaunt with thinning hair.

So far I have thirty-one get-well cards. I hung them in the archway of the living room. Seeing them there brings me joy. Wesley's Uncle Jim and Aunt Charlotte have sent cards signed by their whole family. I appreciate their efforts to show how much they care.

I went to see Dr. McCabe last Monday. He said that it looks like I am doing pretty well, considering. He says I don't have to return to see him unless I want to. I will. I like him to keep an eye on things.

He was upset with me when I told him that I stopped taking my birth control pills the night I found out about the cancer. He said this was no time to be getting pregnant. I told him that we would be careful, but that I didn't want to put those hormones into my body ever again. I had read on the package that the pill could cause gallbladder disease and other complications, so if I already had my gallbladder removed, maybe some of the other risks might affect me as well. He was direct with his disapproval and said that if we weren't careful, we might end up with a baby with one eye in the middle of its forehead from the chemotherapy. I told him to let us worry about that.

I got my period this morning. Dr. Verma had said that I probably wouldn't have one during treatment, but I think I willed it to happen. I feel like as long as that comes, maybe my ovaries will remain intact and we can have a baby one day when all of this has passed.

6:17 P.M.—I won't get to have chemo again tomorrow. My white blood cell count is only 2.4 this time. Dr. Verma said he discussed giving me Neupogen with Dr. McCabe. They agreed it would be beneficial and help get me on the originally scheduled regimen of treatment.

Neupogen is a drug that stimulates the white blood cells to grow and can be used when white blood cell depletion is the only factor delaying treatment. It means I will have to give myself shots every day, but it'll be worth it. Wesley will help me. I won't start the medicine until after my next treatment. I just hope it works.

Thursday, February 22

Lately, Vance and I have been talking on the telephone a lot. It amazes me that he is someone I have come to seek and to find such comfort from. Over the past eight years or more, Vance has been living his life in a way I respect. He lives his life consciously and has grown from the people he chooses to surround himself with. I don't think a woman like Heather would have come to him in the years he spent living more for himself than in the consideration of others. I've watched him grow into man, and I respect him now. He loves his wife, is good to our family, and has a oneness with nature that propels him in a positive way.

I have been telling him about the things I have read about creative visualization and how some cancer patients use it as a tool to visualize the cancer going away. I read about one patient who imagined the chemo being a Pac-Man and the cancer being the little pellets. When the patient had treatment, he would visual the Pac-Man eating up the pellets, thus eating up the cancer. I also read about another woman who visualized the cancer as ice and the chemo as hot water. When the hot water goes in, it melts the ice and flushes out the cancer.

Ever since I first felt the warmth in my chest a few days

after each treatment, I have visualized it melting away. Mary told me I would feel warmth in the area of the tumors a few days into each treatment. I didn't even know about creative visualization. Vance said he would send me a good book on the subject, and I received it today. Within the first two chapters, I was captivated by the possibilities, until I finally had to stop reading and do some writing.

My parents said the other day that they want to throw me a huge "got well" party when this is over, so I have begun to focus on that as the closure we will all receive and deserve when I have completed treatment. I thought deeply about what I visualize that day to be like, and this is what I wrote:

I rise from where I read the words that my brother wanted to share. I don't get far, because I believe the music, the sun and the perfection of feeling so cared about has inspired me to share what I have come to learn in such a short time about people and the mind and the hope for something like a miracle.

It starts with something that changes so much inside of me. I hope for so many things to come to the place that I have found myself in. I hope and believe in things that I am told, things that are written, and most of all, things that I feel. These are things that cannot be seen but are here, even before tragedy and between triumph. I believe, and it will happen. I have faith, and it will come. I see it, and it becomes real.

The day is beautiful as I sit in my room and prepare my appearance for the guests to arrive. They are people who are members of the life I lead and who have somehow inspired me to heal— to want to heal. I sit in front of the mirror wearing a hat that was sewn by the hands of my mother, who is certainly a healer, and I put colors on my face. I am not ashamed. The locks of my hair remain within me but have not yet shown themselves.

My eyes are clear, my clothes fit nicely and the house smells of wonderful foods like zucchini bread and the chicken that grills slowly with my father's concocted sauce. The smells seep into my room as do the sounds of Bob Seger, who I am certain wrote "Roll Me Away" just for me. The music and sounds that I heard as a child and desire as an adult are loud and fun the way our house has always been to me.

My husband showers and meets me in the bedroom, following his usual rituals. He tells me I look beautiful. I see him there, a better man for the husband he has been and a better person for what he has gone through himself. And I am certain a better father one day for knowing what life can offer when having the strength to show his children that tragedies can turn to triumph if you truly believe in and love those you share your life with. I once heard a saying that the best thing a father can do for his children is to love their mother. I believe that is true. I was shown it as a child.

As I prepare for my guests, I am certain it is one of the most important days of my life. It's the day I gather with the people who helped bring me out of the darkness and into the light that carried me through to the place I desired more than just about anywhere else—the safe haven that lets me live a very long time. Not only live long but also live better because I have conquered something that few people my age will ever have to face. I have to say that I have seen God in a way that allows me to thank him for the experience and trust that my time to meet him is still far away. I glimpse into the place of death where people I love have already gone and know that although they wait for us all, they rally for my freedom in the land of the living. They walk with me in spirit and shine light when I need it. They carry me when I am weak, and they, too, believe in me as much as I have come to believe in myself.

My life gets to be something totally new and different than it would have been, because I fought the fight that I was given. And even though the fight can be as simple as getting out of bed one day or as difficult as fighting the fears that treatment brings another, my fight is my own, and by that day I will have fought it well. I will have survived and all that I know can be shared. And all that was at my expense can be taught to others, not really by me, but by each person who chooses to benefit, because though I was stricken, I believe I was chosen to help. All that I endured can be for a reason.

I hug the people I love, and I bask in the reality that what I am there for is to celebrate life, and that will be my moment—when I see those gathered around me in joy and celebration. Those who have agonized with me and sat at the foot of their bed, or stood atop a mountain to talk with their maker about making me well. These will be the guests in my childhood home. There will be much happiness, and the words I share will give me strength in the realization that I have survived. My parents will rest in the knowledge that their desire for their children to outlive them is again possible. My mother's worries will be eased of the fear the medicine brought her. My parents will get to feel good again, as I am certain my illness has brought them much pain.

I have always been a dreamer, dreaming both wonderful and terrible things. All I see in the visions of hope are places of peace, feelings of joy, and the perfection of good health that comes after a journey such as this one. The calm has arrived after a vigorous storm and the shelter I found in the arms, strength and faith of others has lifted me in my greatest time of need. I have arrived home for a while—to learn, to live and to give something back. May the day come that I add to the human race—I pray that it does—it will all become clear that it is a cycle we participate in, and we are all vital participants in that cycle.

Let others realize how much they love me. Let me realize how much I love others. Let all things be better after something bad. Let there be healing, let there be comfort and let there be peace. For we all will have struggled, we all will have triumphed and we all will be better because of it.

That is what I dream today. And as the siren roars outside of my window, I pray for the person that those sirens are heading towards, because I realize we all need to be lifted at times. May we all rise to those who have fallen and share with those in need.

I am thankful to be sitting in my kitchen with my husband preparing a meal and with a friend on the way. On this day, I feel good.

Nine

Tuesday, February 27

7:20 A.M.—I went in for blood work at 6:30 A.M. yesterday morning. The ladies who work at the lab are always so nice to me. Nancy, one of the women who works at the lab, is always talking about her niece who had Hodgkin's and went on to recover and have two children. Children—dear God, let there be children.

My blood work indicated my white blood cell count was 5.32, so Dr. Verma is going to let me go forward with treatment since I will be starting the Neupogen shots with this cycle. I also had a chest X-ray yesterday, but I won't know the results of that until I talk to Dr. Verma later this week. I just pray the chemo has been working.

I have chemo in a few hours. Wesley, my mom, Jeri and Bev are going. Bev had surgery on her knee last week, so she won't be able to be there for very long. I told her she didn't need to go at all, but she insisted.

4:20 P.M.—I keep trying to project how many more treatments I will have to endure, but there is really no way to tell, especially since we still do not have any confirmation that the cycles are working.

Mary talked with me today about the support group that the hospital offers on Tuesday nights. She suggested that I go. I'm really not one for a group setting. Besides, I just don't know why anyone would want to sit amongst so many people who are suffering through cancer. I am apprehensive about going, but I think if I feel up to it, I might go for a little while. If nothing else, it will give me some place to be other than at home. Mary told me about a woman named Kate who also has Hodgkin's and goes to the group meeting. She's forty, which doesn't fit the profile, but she has it nonetheless.

I am supposed to pick up my prescription for Neupogen tomorrow and start the shots on Thursday, but my friend, Kati, called from the pharmacy to say that she was having trouble getting them under my coverage, but she will try and work it out. It scares me to think what will happen if she doesn't, because Dr. Verma went ahead with treatment even though my white count was low. He counted on me getting the Neupogen. I just have to leave this one up to her; otherwise I will drive myself crazy.

Even though the effects after treatment do not seem to be worsening, the effects during treatment are getting more and more difficult. I had to really fight vomiting today when she started my Benadryl and Velban "push." It's called a push when they insert it directly into the IV rather than hanging it in a bag to drip into the tube. I seem to be experiencing every other side effect from treatments and the administering of them, but I have not yet vomited. I continue to fight the urge, even though it would probably make me feel better.

Mary usually orders me lunch during treatment, but I didn't eat any of it today. In fact, I will probably never eat another turkey sandwich or purple grapes again. Even though we are administering the treatment more quickly each time, the process still seems to take forever. I sit and watch the IV drip and wonder how it all works and hope it all works. The Velban still hurts going in. We have tried everything to help alleviate the pain. Mary even read that dimming the lights and putting a dark bag over the drip bag helps. We tried it, and at first it seemed to, but I think that was just wishful thinking. The pain crept up on me and caught me off guard.

"Go get Mary! Go get Mary!" I told Wesley.

He went to get her without asking why. He could see that I was in pain, and the time it took to figure out what was causing it would only make it last longer.

"What's the matter, Lisa?" my mom asked.

"It's burning! Please rub my arm!"

My mom was out of her chair and next to me before I even finished my sentence. Mary rushed in and slowed down the drip. Within seconds it felt better, and I was able to handle the adjusted dose of pain. It was still very painful, but at least it was more manageable.

10:14 P.M.—I went to the support group, although supported is not what I really felt. The first thing I didn't like was that for refreshments they served every kind of caffeine drink there was. I would think they would offer juice or water, given the health many of us were in. I had heard that I wasn't supposed to have carbonated drinks during treatment, but they told me that wasn't true, so I did indulge in one. It tasted like syrup after being away from it for so long.

There were some people there who had been well for several years but kept going to the meetings each week regardless. I can't relate to that. I was the youngest patient there. The people there had all different kinds of cancer—colon, breast, lung and others. There was a young guy named Mike, about thirty years old, who has brain cancer. He had an operation to minimize the tumor, and it doesn't seem to be growing right now. He's trying to avoid chemotherapy at all costs. I was deeply offended by him as soon as he spoke.

"I just don't see how I could let them put that poison into my body. That'll kill me long before this tumor will," Mike said. "That would be the death of me."

I thought that was a pretty bold statement given the company he was in. Did he not look around the room and see those of us who were losing our hair and had the obvious mark of chemo? Did he not care? What stumped me most was that he seemed to feel so much more comfortable with the radiation he had received to his brain than he did about the idea of receiving chemo. I sat there and tried not to judge and that was hard, but it was even harder not to speak in our defense. I somehow managed to remain silent, but it wasn't easy.

I've discovered that there seems to be this trend where people are either for or against Western medicine, chemo specifically. I don't understand it at all. Can't people just be for life and trying to achieve that however possible?

The psychologist, Bernadette, who leads the group, has never had cancer. She started the group on her own several years ago on a voluntary basis. There was also a woman there, Lynn, who videos the meetings for a television project she is working on. She also has never had cancer, and I could tell she was uncomfortable when the circle of conversation came to her, and she was asked how things have been going for her in her life. Could she really complain about work or boast about her love life in a circle of cancer patients? Everyone else there used to have cancer, was still battling it or loved someone who had it.

I wasn't very comfortable there, and when it came my turn to speak I held back.

"Lisa, is there anything you would like to share?" Bernadette asked.

"I have Hodgkin's disease and my nurse, Mary, suggested that I come," I answered.

"Mary Trevor? She's a great nurse," Bernadette responded.

"Yeah, she really is," I agreed. "I just mainly wanted to come and listen. I really am doing fine. I had treatment this morning and am feeling pretty good. Just tired."

"How has this whole experience been impacting your life? Are you able to cope with the fact that you have cancer?" she asked.

Another bold move and question asked by someone who has never had cancer.

"Yeah, I just take it one day at a time. I have my family and that helps. I know I will get better."

She could tell I wasn't interested in divulging how I felt or why I felt that way. She welcomed me to the group and moved on to the next person.

Other people were much more comfortable with sharing. They talked about everything from their ski trips to their catheter infections. I just listened and wondered what made it all tick. What made this group work and how did these people manage to get up every day—just like me? How did any of us manage to get up every day?

A young woman who was just diagnosed with cervical cancer was also visiting the group for the first time. She had just been told two days before, and I recognized the shocked and confused look in her eyes as the same look I had in the early days of my diagnosis. After sharing her diagnosis and prognosis with us, she began to ask questions about how each of us dealt with the news when we were told. She couldn't have been more than ten years older than me, and even though I didn't feel comfortable talking about my own plight, I was happy to try and encourage her in anyway that I could.

"The best thing you can do is just move forward with

doctors that you trust and just find your own pace in dealing with this," I offered.

"But how do I find my pace?" she asked.

"You just wake up every day and find a reason to live. Sometimes it's revealed in more obvious ways than others are, but everyday there is a reason. It's the hardest thing, especially when you are so scared. But with each treatment and test that shows it's working, the belief that you can get well will get stronger and stronger."

She didn't seem convinced. I didn't expect our encouraging words to offer her much comfort right then, but I thought that maybe in the days to come, she might remember the words of the people who have cancer in common with her, and that might be helpful. It was easy for me to coach her to look toward surviving, but it wasn't always easy to believe in the same for myself. Maybe in the days and weeks to come I might also remember the words of encouragement and begin to trust in them.

I doubt I will go to the group meeting again. At least I can say I tried. That should count for something.

Thursday, March 1

7:45 P.M.—Kati worked it all out, and I was able to pick up my Neupogen prescription this morning. Wesley and I went to Dr. Verma's office and one of the nurses showed us how to administer the shots. She used saline on herself and on me. The needle didn't really hurt going in, because it is very sharp and small, but the fluid being pushed out of the needle and into my flesh really stung.

"You need to push the air out of the needle before you begin, choose a spot on your thigh or lower abdomen, squeeze an area of fat and put the needle in at an angle. Then, before you push in the fluid, you need to aspirate slightly to make sure you have not entered a blood vessel and there is no blood. Once you've done that, just push in the medicine, pull out the needle, apply pressure and a Band-Aid, and you're done. Now, you try it," she told me.

"Like this?" I asked, tugging at my leg.

"That's right."

I did everything she said, but when it came time to stick the needle in, I hesitated.

"It's okay. Just take your time," Wesley said.

"You'll see. It doesn't hurt a bit," the nurse said.

I finally worked up the nerve to stick myself and administer the saline. It stung again, but it was easier than I thought.

"And this will keep my white blood cell count up so I can stay on schedule with chemo?" I asked for reassurance.

"It should," the nurse answered.

"It will," Wesley said.

And that's all that really matters. As silly as it sounds, I would let them hit me over the head with a two-by-four if it meant I could be one step closer to getting rid of this cancer. Anything to get rid of the cancer.

The nurse sent me home with instructions for rotating spots that I give myself shots in. Because the shots make my bone marrow work harder to make the good cells, it can sometimes cause me to suffer from minor aches and pains. My friend Darcy's dad, Bob, had these shots when he went through treatment for non-Hodgkin's lymphoma, and her mom said that his legs and back sometimes ached. Janice, Darcy's mom, suggested I give myself the shots in the evening, when I will be more rested, rather than early in the day when I will be exerting more energy and causing my body to work harder to make white blood cells.

We decided that 4:00 P.M. would be the best time to have the shots. I was more nervous about the effect the Neupogen would have on my body than I was about the shot itself. I have never really feared needles, so that made it easier. A little easier.

9:32 P.M.—I spent some of the night on the phone with my mom's lifelong friend Carlita. The most endearing thing about our conversation wasn't the stories she told me of when my mom was a child or what my parents were like when they first married, it was knowing that she would have stayed on the phone with me all night if I needed her to. She put my mind at ease, and I talked with her until I felt better about being home alone.

Of all nights, this was the first that I was left alone. I didn't really choose it, it just happened. Wesley found a part-time janitorial job working early in the morning, but they asked him to work tonight so they could train him. His hours will be ideal once his regular schedule begins, because he will be home from work before I even wake up. That way, on the days I am sick and need his help, he will be here with me instead of at work. He only had to work for a few hours tonight. My mom went to a movie with a friend. I didn't want to go, because I limit myself to weekdays, first-showing movies so I won't be exposed to as many people. Those are two of the rules—no shopping malls and no busy movie theaters. I always follow the rules.

Without realizing it, by declining to go to the movies and insisting that my mother go and enjoy herself, I was forcing myself to be alone. Initially, I waited to see if the shots would take immediate affect and would call for Tylenol, and then I decided to watch some television. I tried and tried to divert my attention to anything but the obvious, and the obvious was that I was still afraid to be alone. It wasn't the fear of a potential prowler or a scary movie on television; it was simply the hard truth of my torment. I find myself in the throes of what this cancer has taken from me, and again I am reminded of what has been lost.

I was the kid who used to tack up my brother's *Star Wars* sheets over the windows where curtains alone did not cover the glare of the outside night and what could be gazing inside. It always unnerved my parents when they would come home and see that I had been up to my tacking of walls, but they never blamed the baby-sitters for permitting it. I was a determined kid, and they knew it was in the best interest of the baby-sitter to humor me. Ironically, I now realize that for all of the times I was afraid of what lurked outside of my home, it was something from inside of me that rocked the very ground I once stood on. What was once a solid foundation below my feet throughout my life was now merely clay. Only my family's protection shielded me from what might have been quicksand.

Just when I think that this whole experience is making me stronger, I realize that what still remains is what has been lost. Can I beg for what once was? Can I ever see things through the eyes of the person I used to be? The more I question, the more I regret the questions, because I know that I can only learn from this what I am open to learning. At the end of all of this pain, there must be joy and triumph waiting to embrace us all. So I am alone for a few hours tonight, can't it just be that everyone else had plans and I was eager for some long-awaited time to myself? Wouldn't any one of them enjoy the same time to be alone with their thoughts? Questions, questions. Before I had to answer with uncertainty, I heard a key turn in the lock of the front door. When it opened, I saw Wesley on its other side. At last, a diversion.

Wednesday, March 6

So far, the shots have been doing their job. I stopped taking the Neupogen on Monday, because my blood count was up to 14, then I started it again when my count plummeted to 2.4 this morning. Dr. Verma said it might take a few weeks to figure out what dose will be necessary for me to maintain a favorable white blood cell count. That's one of the things I have learned about this treatment process: Everyone is different and as much as I'd like for it to be, it's not an exact science.

I got some good news this morning. Dr. Verma called to say that my X-ray showed improvement. It took the first sign of improvement for me to realize it, but Dr. Verma operates with caution and skepticism. He didn't try to diminish my happiness, but I sensed he is a "proceed with caution" kind of man. He says I'll have a CT scan after the fourth treatment. A chest X-ray that showed improvement will get me through until the next milestone is reached.

I went to the support group meeting for the second and final time last night. I wasn't certain I wanted to go, but then I found myself there again. Once again, I left feeling worse than when I arrived and have decided that it's not a place I can go to receive comfort. If there is no comfort in it for me, I do not belong there.

I try not to judge what the others feel about the group and why they continue to go. I know that being just a babe in the woods must force me to miss the big picture that many of them are able to clearly see.

There was a woman there again who was very distraught last week. She told us that her husband would soon die from lung cancer. She talked about how much the group has helped her realize that she has had her "head up her ass." Those were her exact words.

"Excuse me ladies and gentlemen, but it's true," she said. "Coming here has made me see that I have been wasting my time with my anger and rage over losing my husband, so I am going to enjoy my time with him for as long as I have him."

For her, I can understand why the group works, and I

could see the difference in her from one week to the next. She sought and found solace there, and if that makes it easier for her in these last days with her husband, then the group has served its purpose for her.

Mike was at group and was talking negatively again. Listening to him speak about his brain tumor and the impact it had on his life, I realized that I was feeling a sense of guilt that carried over from last week. I sat there and listened to others talk about their cancer experiences and I felt guilty for being the one with the most treatable form. It made me question whether or not I even had a right to be there. Does a person with my statistics for survival have the right to feel so sad when there are others with worse plights?

I stopped questioning it the more I listened to Mike talk about himself. I just kept getting so irritated with the whole group.

"I keep thinking about my children and how they will not remember me. It just doesn't seem fair," he explained.

I wondered to myself if I had missed something from the week before. Wasn't this the same guy who had said that the tumor wasn't growing and that radiation was working? Why these negative thoughts now?

"Oh sure your children will remember you. You're their father," Bernadette said.

Other members of the group kept interjecting their words of encouragement, but I kept wondering why no one was saying the complete opposite. Over and over again, I kept hearing the same thing, until finally I had to speak up.

"Mike, you could very well survive this. You could beat this cancer and raise your own children," I interjected.

Quiet came over the room, and Mike looked at me along with the others. I am sure he had considered that possibility, but he must have gotten sidetracked, because he looked at me like it was something he hadn't thought about—at least for a very long time. He didn't really reply but looked at me in a way that made me feel better for saying it.

I almost felt badly for saying anything at all, because I only know what it's like to have Hodgkin's disease and travel my own fate. I cannot presume to understand the torment of knowing there is something that may or may not be growing recklessly in my brain. I just wanted him to remember that miracles do occur every day, and it's not over until it's over. Will his kids have their father to raise them? No one can tell him that. But is it possible? Yes, and someone should remind him of that from time to time.

As I listened to the rest of the group speak, I just kept saying to myself, "How did I end up here? How did I end up here?" The question kept repeating inside of my head, until finally tears began to well up in my eyes. And that was right about the time it came my turn to speak.

"Lisa, how are you doing tonight?" Bernadette asked.

"I'm fine. I'm doing fine," I answered.

She looked at me for a moment, then proceeded further.

"Are you doing okay? You look like you have something you want to say," she continued.

"I . . . I," I tried to find the words to explain my anguish. "I am just looking around the room and listening to these words about cancer, and with all of my heart I cannot believe I am here. How did I end up here?"

"What do you mean?" she asked.

"I mean, I'm twenty-four years old. I can't begin to imagine sitting in this room a few years from now. I just have to move forward. I have to get well and never return to what brought me here. To this place in my life . . . I'm only twenty-four," I said as the well of tears left my eyes and ran down my cheeks.

"You're not talking about this group, are you Lisa?" she assumed.

"No. I have cancer. And I'm just trying to figure out when

I went from the person I was to the person who sits in a room telling everyone about how great things are going, despite the fact that I have cancer. I don't belong here," I tried to explain.

"And you just want to get well and move on with your life and try to put it all behind you—like it never happened?" she asked.

"No, like it will never happen again."

She smiled something warm and reassuring at me, and in that instant I accepted them all as soldiers in the same battle I was fighting, but I decided I could not return to the group. I wasn't strong enough, and I knew I wasn't going to get any stronger there.

Ten

Monday, March 11

I just got home from my appointment with Dr. Verma. He has scheduled a CAT scan following my next treatment. I am anxious and afraid to know how my body is responding to the treatments.

Lately, I have been having difficulties giving myself the shots. Wesley is always there to help me get the needle ready and to hold my skin while I stick myself, but I never let him insert the needle or its contents. The needle doesn't hurt, but the medicine does, so I like to regulate how quickly it goes in.

On Sunday, I couldn't manage to stick myself for some reason. We followed our usual rituals, but when it came time to stick the needle into my leg, I hesitated.

"What are you doing?" Wesley asked.

"I don't know. I just can't do it," I answered.

"Do you want me to do it?"

"No, I have to do it myself," I told him. I was determined to do it just as I had been doing all along.

Several minutes had passed when I started to break out in a sweat.

"Your hands are shaking. Why don't you just let me do it?" Wesley asked again.

"Because I have to do it myself," I repeated, fearing that if I lost control over my ability to do that, other strengths might later weaken.

"Then do it," he replied.

As hard as I tried, I couldn't do it. I would start to stick myself, but then I would stop just as I got the needle next to my skin. Before I knew it, twenty minutes had passed.

"Okay, maybe you should do it, but I don't want you to push the medicine in," I finally agreed.

I reminded him to insert it at an angle to avoid any veins in my leg, and then I handed him the needle.

"Okay, so I just push it in?" he asked. I could tell he was starting to get nervous.

"It'll go in easily. Do it on the count of three." I told him.

"Okay. One. Two. Three," he said, but then he hesitated before inserting it.

"What are you doing?" I asked him, laughing at his nervousness now.

"Okay, I'll do it now," he said, but then he removed the needle as quickly as he inserted it.

"What are you doing?" I asked him. "Why did you do that?"

"I don't know. I thought it would be harder to stick in than it was." By then, we were both laughing.

"I would rather stick myself once than have you stick me twice."

The small prick of the needle made me bleed a little, so we cleaned my leg up and sterilized an area on my other leg. We eventually got it done. Wesley has had to insert the needle every time since that day, but I still push in the medicine.

I have my fourth chemo treatment tomorrow. I get a bit of anxiety before going each time. It's difficult to have something administered that I know is going to make me sick, but I try to stay focused on the big picture.

Wesley's job is going well. He gets up early and goes and is usually back before I even wake up. He doesn't enjoy doing janitorial work, but he never complains to me about it. He gets the job done, so he can get back home to me.

He's getting excited about his trip back to Texas for his brother's wedding. I still wish I could go, but I do not want to risk getting sick and delaying treatment. I am, however, planning a trip to the Bay area to visit my cousin, Corinee, and her family. It's about five hours from here. My grandma is going with me. I don't want to sit around here while Wesley is gone. I will be going the weekend before my fifth treatment, so I shouldn't be feeling too badly, although I don't know how I will manage giving myself shots while he is gone.

I continue to visit websites on the Internet that have stories of other cancer patients, particularly the website set up by a young physician who was diagnosed with Hodgkin's disease. Her website has direct links to other cancer sites. I have read stories of many other Hodgkin's patients and found it helpful. I enjoyed reading of people who have recovered and gone on to live healthy, productive lives. I read of one young man who also suffered the same horrible itching. He went to several doctors and was being treated for allergies for weeks until he was finally diagnosed. The itching started in his feet just like mine.

The get-well cards keep pouring in. I have over forty now and keep encouraging people to send more. The archway to the living room is getting quite full. I've decided that when all of this is over and we have my got-well party, I will invite everyone who sent me a card—and then some.

Tuesday, March 12

11:14 A.M.—It's two hours after my treatment, and I am not feeling well. Treatment was more taxing physically than mentally today. I had to hold back from vomiting during the drug that made me itch. I am told that I am probably halfway through treatment now, and I am certain my body is aware of it. The feelings I get in my stomach remind me of how serious all of this is and what a toll it is taking on my body. Though my spirit remains strong, sometimes my body gets weak.

I realize that even with a good CAT scan, there are to be many sunrises and sunsets before I reach the end of this journey. I haven't cried a river of tears or sat in a room alone long enough to get extremely sad. It all comes and goes. The sadness is here now, but I know it will pass. The tears I could cry would be tears that I'd waste in place of joy. The joy is coming.

I know God is watching over me. He was with me in my bedroom at night. And he was with me when I was a child and climbed up in the trees to talk with him about things that frightened me and in my car when I used to drive down the country roads to my home and back. He has been with me for as long as I can remember, and he is with me now. He joins me in my childhood room again, where I now sleep with my husband.

I know there is love all around me. I see it in the faces of others, who I know look at me with such pity. I'm someone they have always known with something they have always feared.

It seems strange to me most of the time that it is inside of me—the cancer. I know I didn't invite it to come, but little by little it began to invade space inside of my body, and of all places, beside my heart. It took up space and made other cells cause me to itch, then my chest got full and things began to go wrong. Things began to feel differently. Sickness appeared that I ignored, then a lump appeared that I could not.

I know I still have moments when the fog is a shelter for me. If I realized every moment of every day that I had cancer, my mind would be mush, I am certain. But I remain trusting in the possibility of my survival, and I feel peace in the times that I pray for it. Mostly, I am just praying to be lifted out of the place I have found myself. Let me be removed from this time in my life when cancer is leering at every turn. I want to be carried out of this place of sickness that I have known for only a short time and returned to the place I spent most of my life where there was good health, peace and trust in the body I was given.

I wait. I wait patiently and know that God's timing is perfect. I've seen it so many times. Sometimes the timing is perfect in small ways but also in vast ways that I remember. Like when I got to my grandpa in time before he died to sit beside him and ask him if he knew God would take care of him. I got to lay next to him and hear what would be his last breaths and know that I was seeing him out of this life and into the next.

There was the time we drove all the way from Texas to California to spend the last day of Alton's life with him, to watch football with him, and to tell him we loved him every time we entered or left his hospital room.

It's these times that helped shape my life and taught me to believe that God was merciful. As he takes one life, he changes another. And now I am again blessed with his timing. I am blessed because I was sitting in the office of the doctor who delivered me, and I went home to parents who loved me, and I felt loved by the man who married me. I don't invite the self-pity that could come with a disease like this one. I know in what ways I am fortunate, and I welcome the things that help lift me during this difficult time.

I have the love of the parents he chose for me, and I know in the deep corners of their hearts they probably cry every day for what I have to go through and wish it were they instead. But that is what good parents do, and that's what I've always known.

There is also the brother that God gave to me when he gave my parents their son. And though it took years for us to really love each other, he's someone who I am lucky to share the blood that runs through my veins. I know that is an important lesson I have learned through the years I have accumulated as an adult. I know that when he reaches the top of a mountain he has me with him. And when it's safe to stop thinking about what he has to do, he thinks of me, his sister. And now I know he loves me more than he ever thought he could. I know we are given in our lives people who are supposed to help us through the experiences that life offers. And of all the people I am blessed to know, it is his presence and his guidance in my life that leads me to faraway places I would have never sought or found without him. And the woman he chose didn't realize her wisdom when she sent me the card that said what my new path represented, "There is no way to peace, Peace is the way."

And there's my husband—the boy I've watched grow into a man, the person I've known most of my life and loved all of that time. I made choices long ago that I know saved me from a life that would have never allowed me all that I experience today geographically, mentally, physically and spiritually. Loving him has helped me to become whole in that our love has endured, and I have truly learned to love unconditionally. Sometimes I have learned the hard way, but the lessons I am still grateful for. I now revel in the love that I know God intended for me to experience. I know loyalty and passion, and I have been lucky enough to watch a person realize how much he is loved, which can be a wonderful thing after a life of not always feeling it even though it was there all of the time.

The rest are people who brighten my days, and it is the way God intended. It's the love of my family that helps me to endure. It is the kindness of all that get me through a day. And though some lights shine brighter than others, they all offer light at the end of my tunnel.

I wait patiently for the mercies of my maker and pay close attention to what happens to others and me because of this. It is during these moments that I wish I could sit with my grandpa and talk with him about what changed us both. I know he'd be angry because the same thing that invaded his body also invaded mine.

During these moments I miss him more than I have missed him in a long time. I sit and think about the impact his illness had on me and although he was accepting of the cancer, I know there must have been times when he watched us all and wished he could stay.

When I sit amongst our family, I think of the times we gathered just for him. Although the cells that mutated in me will soon be gone and allow me to recover, heal and survive, I feel as he must have sometimes, and I wonder how it all went wrong inside. When I am tired and sick, I think of the times I saw him sitting with his face in his hands and now recognize the agony of it.

I still wish I could sit with him to speak about the strange bond we share. I could tell him what I feel and, even though it wasn't the same cancer, maybe I could share this with someone that loved me and feel the validation that a support group or a loving card cannot offer.

Wednesday, March 13

Wesley and Amber's sister Amy have a birthday today. Occasions like this make Wesley miss his father even more, especially the years he remembers being close to him as a child. I think that much of what I felt for Wesley in the early years that I knew him was something that would take years for me to completely understand. Some people tend to be the rescuers of others in different life experiences, and although I was too young and too separate from him at the young age we met, I must have sensed his sorrow for what had come to his life with his parents' divorce. I guess I would have wanted to try and rescue him if I were capable.

Even at that young age, or especially at that young age, I knew Wesley had something different than I did, and his existence seemed to be a bit of a mystery to me. He has called my family the apple pie American family, but we all have since realized that we were really nothing of the sort. But what we were and still are is a family that, to this day, remains committed to our togetherness, which is one of the things Wesley has continued to admire.

I spent much of my childhood putting Wesley and the image I had of him in a safe place for me to keep only for myself. Years passed between the times we would see each other, but still, the feelings I had for him remained within me. Until finally, as I grew older and became more than the girl who used to live down the street from him, he began to see in me the possibilities of a love that he still thinks is among the purest things he has ever received in life. My parents may have thought that I would eventually come to realize that Wesley was not all that I had built him up to be in that place I reserved just for him inside of my heart, but I could never be convinced of that. And so finally, I set out to find what I had always been looking for, and I found him. And in the years that Wesley and I have been together, I think my parents have realized that Wesley was right for me all along. There is something to be said for following your heart to find true happiness, because no one should ever settle for a love less than wonderful. It's a lesson that many learn the hard way, but the lesson learned is what is important.

After Wesley's father died more than a year ago, he wouldn't talk about it unless he was drinking, which only made it worse. Our relationship suffered for months because of it, until last August when he finally decided to stop drinking so he could come to terms with his father's death and all the hurt that came with it. Over the past several months he'd managed to make sense of many things that had been left unanswered when his father died. With our relationship intact, we were able to move beyond the pain and discover a new side of ourselves.

Tuesday, March 19

I keep willing my menstrual cycle to come each month, believing that it will better my chances for having children later. My will is strong. It came again today and has every twenty-eight days since this all began. Thank God for small miracles.

I have been going to the lab several times a week while Dr. Verma regulates my shots. During my last set of labs, he discovered that my potassium was too low, so he prescribed a potassium supplement for me. I have to take it in liquid form for seven days. I only have to take one and a half teaspoons a day, but they taste terrible. I get sick to my stomach enough without having to add to my illness, but I remain ever compliant and have confidence in the decision I made to trust the doctors who have done nothing but good for me thus far.

Wesley leaves on Friday for Wayne's wedding. I am leaving for Corinee's on Thursday. My mom will take Wesley to the airport since he is flying out of Redding. I didn't want to be here when Wesley left. It's always easier to leave than it is to get left. I don't even want to think about the days that he will be gone. I am just happy that he is able to be there to share in his brother's happiness. Wesley is nervous about giving the toast as the best man, but I'm sure the words will come to him.

I am scheduled for a CAT scan on Thursday. I just keep praying for the best.

Tuesday, March 26

Dr. Verma got the results back from my CAT scan and said that the test showed "dramatic response." He said it was the best-case scenario! To have word that the chemo is working makes all of this worth it. I have said from the beginning that I'll do it all if it means I will get better and never have to go through this again.

Wesley has been gone for four days and it seems my resolve has weakened yet again in his absence. I enjoyed seeing my cousin Corinee and her family over the weekend, but being away from home made me miss Wesley even more. Corinee helped me with my shots and said it was something she would never forget. I guess it's good that she got to see a little bit of what I go through, even if the shots pale in comparison to the rest.

I went to chemo and had the usual people there with me to help get me through it. Everything was the same, and I followed the same pattern as last time by getting sicker as the treatment wore on. I fought the urge to vomit, my hand burned with pain from the Velban, and I passed on the invitation for lunch. Everything seemed to be the same, but it wasn't until Mary spoke her words of wisdom, that I realized why the routine of treatment did not seem so routine and the unfamiliar tears that accompanied it were just my longing coming to the surface.

When I was almost done with my last IV drip, Mary looked at me in a way I rarely see from her. She always has a face of compassion, but on this day, she had a face that fought hard to hide her sadness.

I had been crying off and on toward the end, and nothing seemed to lift my spirits for long when Mary turned to me as she was walking out the door and said, "This one is almost over. He'll be here for the next one."

When she spoke those words, it was like a light went on inside of me, both to show me what I had been lacking and to invite a bit of hope to what had been a more difficult day than most.

I looked at her in a way that expressed my thanks for her observation and almost as if I was asking a question, I said, "That's why I'm having such a hard day?"

"Next time will be easier," she said softly.

My mom and Bev both looked at me and smiled. I finally felt free to let the tears fall. I realized I wasn't crying only because I was growing weary of the treatments, but I was also crying because Wesley was gone and everything seemed harder without him. I cried and cried, then smiled in between. And suddenly, I felt lucky for what had come to me in that brief moment between the pain and the sickness that accompanied such a day, and I knew that with Wesley, all things were more bearable.

Eleven

Monday, April 1

I have been counting the days, and now the hours, until Wesley comes home. He'll be back tomorrow. I am so relieved. I enjoyed my visit with Corinee and her family, but I was even more lonely there than at home without Wesley. I watched their everyday lives and how effortlessly they lived them, and it made me long for the time when Wesley and I lived that way, too. I thought that getting out of town would be helpful. I thought maybe it would be good to get away from it all, but I didn't get away. It followed me there. It follows me everywhere.

I have been spending a lot of time with my cousin Darla. She is ten years older than I am, so we were never really close before now. She'd been living in Hawaii for most of her adult life and has only been back home for a few years. I like to think that one of the blessings I have been given through this experience is my newfound relationship with her. Darla has been helpful to me since this all began and has made time for me even when her young daughter, Tati, was also demanding of her time. I will always be grateful to her and the others for being at chemotherapy with me whenever possible.

Wesley said the wedding went off without a hitch. I got to talk with everyone during the reception. They called me from Wesley's hotel room. I even talked with Wayne and Tara. Wayne said that it was a beautiful day. He had been very nervous in the days leading up to it, but he sounded genuinely happy that it went so well and that he was now married to Tara. He was sweet enough to say again how much he wished I were there. It was a difficult day for me to think about them all there together, because I wished I could have been there. But I was able to feel joy for them and know that their special day turned out as they hoped it would.

My dad left this morning, after being here for three days. He switched weekends and started coming home on the weekend after treatment, because my mom told him he needs to see what really goes on. He didn't really comprehend the difficulties of treatment, because he was coming home just before the next one, after I had a chance to recover and rejuvenate. I felt badly for getting angry with him while he was here, but I just couldn't hide how badly I was feeling to make him feel more at ease.

I woke up on Saturday morning feeling terrible. I had been awake for about an hour, but I was too weak to get out of bed right away. The smell of breakfast cooking in the kitchen was making me feel even worse, so I decided to wait until I was sure my parents were done eating. Just then, my dad knocked on the door and entered with a plate of food.

"Here you go, hon. I made you some breakfast," he said as he set the plate on the bedside table. Before I could thank him, even though I wasn't going to eat, he had already shut the door and was heading back toward the kitchen.

I waited a few more minutes before I went to the kitchen, where I found my mom washing dishes and my dad reading the newspaper. I sat down at the table and just took a minute to collect myself, because the smell of the food was still taunting my stomach.

"Good morning, honey," my dad said in his cheerful voice.

"Good morning," I replied.

"How are you feeling?" my mom asked. "Do you need a nausea pill?"

"I took one before I got out of bed," I answered. I was resting my head on the table when my dad spoke to me again.

"Well, it's a beautiful day outside. Why don't you get dressed and go for a walk? The fresh air will do you some good," my dad said.

My mom turned and looked at him, and without even saying a word, I got up and walked back to my room. In my frustration, I slammed the door behind me. I could hear my dad asking what he'd done wrong.

"Mick, it's not what you did, it's what you said," my mom informed him.

"What? I just thought some fresh air would make her feel better."

"Lisa is very good at doing what she can on the days she feels her worst, and if she comes out here in her robe and rests on the couch all day long, then that's the most she can do. Fresh air won't fix how badly she feels in the first days after a treatment," my mom explained.

"Well, how was I supposed to know that Carmen?" he asked. "I just didn't realize . . ."

"That's why I wanted you home. Now you know," she said.

I couldn't hear them talking anymore, but I could tell she had probably given him a hug. I waited a little while before going back out into the kitchen, and when I did, my dad apologized.

"I'm sorry, Lisa. I just don't know how to project anything

but a positive attitude toward you. I just wish you could feel well and do the things you like to do," he explained.

"I know, Dad. Soon I will be able to," I said, then gave him a hug.

I felt badly for what he was going through, but it wasn't my job to make him feel more comfortable with what was going on. He was going to have to come to terms with it the way the rest of us have.

Giving myself the shots while Wesley has been gone is difficult, especially since my mom is unable to help me. She just can't bear to do any of it. The first day I had to have shots after he left, my mom said I was going to have to figure out a way to do it without her, because she couldn't do it. She offered to call Carlita, but I eventually did it on my own.

My dad helped me with my shots while he was here. He was very nervous at first, especially about the air bubbles that sometimes form from the medicine. I had to convince him that I wasn't going to die from the air bubbles by explaining to him what Mary said about it taking more than a few feet of air in a tube going directly to my vein to cause any problems. He made me get rid of the air bubbles before inserting the needle anyway.

Many people fear needles. I never have. I don't know why I was not able to give myself the shots for a time. Corinee told me how brave I was while I was there. She saw in my face how difficult the shots were for me. I never really thought of any of this process and my ability to cope with it as bravery. I just thought of it as something I had to deal with, because there was no other alternative.

The other day, when I was in Dr. Verma's office, I kept expressing my concern about the chemotherapy and the toll it was taking on my body. I was asking a lot of questions and apologizing for doing so. He said, "I never mind you asking questions as long as you understand the answers."

I questioned what effect the treatments must be having on the rest of my body if it was causing me to lose my hair. I questioned whether I would be able to have children after this was over and if having my period, even though he told me I probably wouldn't, was a good sign. He waited for me to ask each question, and then he walked a few steps closer to me before he spoke.

"Lisa, we warned you of the possibilities and risks before we began," he said.

"I know, but now that it is happening to me, I am getting scared of the risks. What about when we start radiation? What will happen to me then? How will my body possibly be able to recover from that?" I questioned him further.

"All of these are legitimate concerns, but let's again consider the alternative. You have chosen this as your course of action against the cancer, right?"

"Yes, I have."

"And you still believe that this treatment regimen can get rid of your cancer?"

"Yes," I answered.

"What do you think would happen to you without these treatments—if you chose to do nothing?" he asked.

I paused for a moment and thought about what my answer truly meant. I sighed and responded, "I would die."

Dr. Verma placed his hand on my shoulder and said, "And if the treatment works?"

"I live."

I smiled at him and decided then that I would try not to question what I had already chosen, and I would move forward with the faith and the hope that I began this journey with. I left his office feeling stronger than when I arrived.

As I drove home, I kept thinking about Dr. McCabe and wondered if he had realized what a wonderful thing he had done by sending me to Dr. Verma. And for the rest of the day,

I said few words and felt secure in the choices I had made. It was a day of renewal and a day that was needed to help restore my faith in the process that had such taxing elements.

Monday, April 8

Wesley got home safe and sound on Tuesday. My mom left on Saturday to visit my dad. I think she needed some time with him as much as Wesley and I needed time alone. Things have been getting better with the three of us here. We finally decided that it was best to send Huck to stay with Wesley's mom in Texas. I hated to see him go, but after he started chewing off the siding on the back of the house, I realized that having him here was not best. I told Wesley, "Well, when he starts eating the house, it's time for him to go."

My parents paid to have him flown to Texas. I woke up the morning Wesley took him to the airport and said good-bye. He didn't seem to mind leaving. He was just excited about getting in the car. I hoped, if nothing else, my mom felt better about leaving to be with my dad since she didn't have to worry about our dog and the damage Huck might be doing here.

We had a fun weekend. Even though the treatments have been getting harder, the week following treatment I usually feel pretty well. Wesley and I bought some used tennis rackets and started playing at the courts on the golf course where my parents are members. I can't play for very long, but it feels good to be out doing something. Wesley said he is proud of me for pushing myself to do so much in the time that my body allows it.

My friend Lora let me borrow her Rollerblades. I skated all the way to the clubhouse the other day and ate a sandwich. I enjoyed the sandwich, but what little conversation I had with the golf pro Mark, who I have known for only a few years, only made me mad.

I was talking to Mark, answering his questions about the cancer and how my treatment was going, when he showed me, as a few others have before him, that some people just don't get it. He would have been better off not saying anything at all.

"When I finish treatment, I will have more than an 85 percent chance of complete and total remission," I finished explaining to him.

"Yeah, but what if it comes back?" he asked.

I thought that was a stupid question to ask someone in my predicament, but I answered him anyway. "Well, that's why I'll be going in for checkups. I like to think of it as if I will be watched so closely that I will be better off than people who have no idea what is going on inside of their bodies will. Besides, a 15 percent chance of it returning is not very large," I tried telling him.

"Yeah, but that's still a chance. And that's scary!" he said.

I had to wonder what he was thinking to have said such things to me about something he knew so little about. Did he not know how long it took me to convince myself that the statistics I was speaking of offered me enough hope to get me through until I was strong enough to believe in them? Did he not know that every morning when I woke up, cancer was my first thought, always followed by a cloud of question of how this would all turn out? And if he was not capable of realizing these things, because cancer had never lived at his house, couldn't he have just been compassionate enough to either say an encouraging word or say nothing at all?

Before he even finished speaking, I made up my mind that I wasn't going to let him spoil my day or make me question whether or not a 15 percent chance was enough, because I had already made up my mind that it was. For the first time in days, I felt like my body was hungry enough for the sandwich I had just enjoyed, and for the first time in months my body was strong enough to carry me on Rollerblades from my home to the clubhouse. I wasn't about to let him ruin that for me.

I didn't even reply, I just gave him a look that, had he been thinking, might make him think twice before saying something like that to me again. Then, I got up and skated home.

On Sunday, we went to Tom and Jeri's house for Easter. Everyone was waiting for my Uncle Steve to arrive. It was his fiftieth birthday, and he rode his bike more than 250 miles over the past week to get there. He is an avid bicycle rider and wanted to accomplish that ride for his birthday. He arrived on schedule and was beaming with perspiration and pride.

The weekend was fun. I got to see members of our family who live out of town, all of whom are excited to come back for my got-well party when treatment is over. I still don't know when that will be, but I just keep hoping I will finish soon.

Last week, about eight days after treatment, I kept feeling like I might have heartburn or something, because my chest felt very warm. I couldn't figure out what it was, then it suddenly came to me as I was getting dressed.

"Wesley! Wesley!" I called to him from our bedroom as I began walking toward the back door.

"What? What's wrong?" he asked as he met me at the door. "Is everything okay?"

"Yes! Everything is great!" I answered, as he looked puzzled. "Everything is perfect! I figured out what is wrong with my chest and why it feels hot."

"What is it?" he asked.

"Remember how Mary said that I would feel heat in the areas where the cancer was? She said I would feel warmth in the days after treatment."

"Yeah," he said.

"Well, that's what it is. After the first treatment, my entire chest felt hot, but then during the following treatments I didn't pay much attention to the warmth because I was concentrating on other side effects. Well, that's what this is. It's not a little bit of heartburn, it's just that there's so little cancer left that only a small spot in the middle of my chest feels warm."

"Could that really be it, Lisa?" Wesley asked.

"That's exactly what it is. Now that I think about it, the areas of warmth have been getting smaller and smaller each time! That means it's going away. The cancer really is going away!" I exclaimed as I hugged Wesley.

After a long embrace, Wesley said, "It's good to see you smile. You're getting better, Lisa."

"Yes, I am!"

Thursday, April 11

Tuesday was my sixth treatment, and it was definitely the hardest. Darla could not go because Tati was sick. Bev didn't go either, because she couldn't find a baby-sitter for Spencer. He had come with her a few times, but she started leaving him at home after he asked Mary to bring him some chocolate milk. He didn't understand that bringing me food and beverages was the least of her job responsibilities and certainly didn't require her to bring the others anything. She just did it to be nice. Of course I couldn't blame him, because he is only four years old.

I spoke with Jeri last night about Krystal going to my treatment since she was on spring break from school. Krystal had wanted to go, but now that she had the opportunity, she was getting scared. Jeri said that after she told her parents she didn't want to go, she came back out to the family room and said she was going after all.

"Are you sure? Because you don't have to go, you can stay

here with Grandma," they told her.

"I'm sure," she answered, then went back to her bedroom.

I questioned whether or not it was the kind of place an eight-year-old child should be, but Tom and Jeri have never sheltered their children from the realities of the world, and I trusted that they knew what was best for their daughter. At lease when Bev brought Spencer to chemo, he was more interested in cartoons and coloring. I knew Krystal would pay close attention to what was going on.

This treatment was definitely the most physically difficult. Wesley and I were there alone during the first half an hour. Jeri said she decided to wait and let things get going before bringing Krystal in, so she wouldn't have to see me cry when Mary started my IV. I was glad she waited, because the beginning was ugly. There's really no other word for it.

My veins were getting so tough from the chemotherapy that I could hear my vein make a popping sound when the needle entered my hand. Mary tried to find a path of entry that had not been used before, because I told her that my hands were still getting sore in the days following treatment. She did her best.

I'd spent most of the last three treatments carrying an ice pack with me everywhere I went, because the pain and inflammation was so intense. There were a few nights that I was so tired, but I could not sleep because of the pain. I sat up on the couch and cried, begging for mercy so I could just get even a little bit of rest. I wanted to prevent that from happening again if I could.

When Mary administered the Decadron, the anti-nausea drug that made me itch, I immediately felt like I was going to vomit. In the two treatments previous, I had asked for a trash bag but was able to hold back the vomiting. This time, however, I could not.

While I vomited, Wesley held the trash bag for me and

Mary put a cold cloth on my forehead. Wesley was so help-ful that I almost forgot what a weak stomach he had. In between the vomiting, tears fell from my eyes.

"Please make it stop. Please make it stop," I said, although not really speaking to either of them specifically.

"Maybe this will be the last one," Mary said.

"It has to be," I said. The vomit was yellow, burned com-ing up and lacked any remnants of food, because I was again feeling too ill to eat in the days before. The treatments were taking their toll again and again. It was over. It had to be. My body was done—no more chemo.

Jeri arrived with Krystal after things had calmed down. Krystal has never been a very shy kid, but she kept to herself and sat close to her mom while she was there. I tried talking with her and setting her at ease, but she still seemed uncom-fortable. They stayed less than an hour. I was actually as relieved as Krystal when she left, because I didn't have the energy to try and look like the treatment wasn't difficult.

I just kept praying that it would be the last one. Dr. Verma told me that he was going to order another gallium scan after this treatment to decide if we should go further with chemotherapy. Throughout treatment, I remembered Dr. Verma telling me in the beginning that this treatment regi-men called for either three or six cycles, each cycle consist-ing of two actual treatments. How many cycles I would have to endure depended on how well my body responded to the first three. I kept trying to imagine myself going back six more times, and the thought overwhelmed me. I would have to have three more cycles of this regimen, because it was all or nothing. I was praying for the latter. My body could not take anymore.

About halfway into treatment, the phone rang. It was Kim calling from Dr. Verma's office. They had scheduled a gallium scan for Thursday and wanted to know if that was okay with me. Mary covered the phone and asked me what I wanted to do.

"I don't want to have the test on Thursday," I told her.

"You're probably not going to feel up to it by then," she said.

"Not only that, but if I have the test so soon then this treatment won't have a chance to do its work. If it means more treatment or the end of treatment based on this test, then I want to give it every opportunity to work before getting tested. What should I do?" I asked her.

"You can do whatever you want. You don't have to go just because they scheduled it. You can have them reschedule it for whenever you want," she answered.

It had never occurred to me before that I had an option to choose not to go when they asked. So I said, "Tell them to wait until next week."

She told them to reschedule, and they did with no questions asked. I'm going in next Wednesday.

After the phone call, I changed my focus and started trying to think positively that I would not have to return for more chemo. And as the red Adriamycin dripped slowly from the bag and into my body, I told myself that it was the last time I would have to watch the drugs trickle into my veins—no more cancer, no more chemo. There was no other alternative.

Treatment finally ended, and Wesley took me home. When we arrived, the house felt quiet and empty. I felt quiet and empty. We spent most of the day on the couch. I didn't even eat until Wednesday morning. I slept most of the next day. I needed the rest. I wanted to give my body the chance it needed to heal. I was asking a lot of my body to give me what I wanted, but I remained in constant prayer—no more cancer, no more chemo.

I called Krystal during the evening after treatment. I didn't know that Jeri was listening on the phone line while Krystal and I spoke.

"Krystal, I just wanted to call and make sure you were okay with what went on today at the hospital. I wondered if you had any questions you might want to ask me," I said to her.

"No, I don't think I do," she replied.

"You're sure?" I asked.

"Yeah, I think so."

We talked for a few more minutes, and then we said goodbye. I started to hang up the phone, but then I heard Jeri's voice. Krystal had not hung up the phone properly.

"Krystal, you should have asked her what you were asking me when we left today," Jeri told her.

"Well, I didn't know what to say," she said.

"Get back on the phone and call her. She won't mind answering your questions," Jeri said.

I heard Krystal say she would, so I hung up the phone and waited for her to call me back. She did.

"Um, Lisa?" she said softly.

"Yes, Krystal," I answered.

"I do have a few questions about today."

"Okay. What do you want to ask me?"

"Well, I was wondering what that red stuff was that was in the bag and was going into your hand. How come it was red?" she asked.

"I don't know why it's red, but that is a medicine that will help the cancer go away."

"Did it hurt?" she asked.

She wasn't there for the drug that made my arm burn. "No, it doesn't hurt at all. Do you have any other questions," I asked her further.

"Mom, did I have any other questions?" I heard her ask Jeri as she covered the phone. "Oh yeah. How come you were shaking like that? Were you cold?"

"Yes. The medicine gives me the chills sometimes while it is going into my hand. That's why Mary gave me warm blankets."

"Well, okay. I think that's all I wanted to know."

"Okay. Krystal?" I said.

"Yeah," she answered.

"Thanks for going today."

"You're welcome."

I hung up the phone and felt good for having talked with her. Jeri called me back right away and thanked me for calling. Jeri started to cry and said that it meant a lot to Krystal to go and that she hoped her being there had made me feel better. She told me that when they left the hospital, Krystal started crying in the car. She thought I was shaking during treatment because I was in pain. Jeri explained it to her, but it made Krystal feel better hearing it from me.

Tuesday, April 16

I am feeling better today. It took all weekend for my body to recover from treatment. I started my period again yesterday. And again, I wonder if I am asking too much of myself for what is ahead.

I got a card from my friend Tanya today. With it, she sent me the book, *The Cancer Conqueror*. I read it front to back already. The book was fascinatingly written by a man who had terminal lung cancer and was told he had only one month to live. He lived beyond that month and ended up ridding himself of the cancer, with the help of conventional treatment, after going to see a man he called The Cancer Conqueror.

Within the book, the man wrote about what causes our bodies to grow cancerous cells, and not just biologically but also emotionally and spiritually. He listed numerous personality traits that many cancer patients have in common, and I was amazed to read that I fit most of them at the time I was diagnosed and in the few years before. It said that many people who get cancer have lived their life in judgment of others and have had a need for extra attention in their life. The words that I was reading were like an awakening to me. I had lived my life that way and in many of the other ways that were listed. The book said that we have the power to actually will cancer to happen. That if we tell our bodies something enough times then it can become true. Just like when we think about a lemon and our mouth begins to water. Our bodies don't always know the difference between what we are telling it and what is actually the truth for it.

I thought about all of the times that I feared getting cancer or another illness as a child. I couldn't imagine how my body could get me through adolescence without getting sick. I thought about the girl in grade school who had hair like mine is now. How many times did I question the capabilities of my body? And by doing that, how many times did I taunt it to do what I was truly asking of it?

I began to think about when I was a child and wanted a broken arm so I could get attention at home and at school and have everyone sign my cast. I remembered the times when all of the yeast infections began when the cancer had started growing and I didn't know it. One nurse practitioner said that maybe I had diabetes and should have a blood test, because she thought maybe the birth control I was taking was a contributing factor. Why didn't that devastate me? I think that I figured diabetes wasn't the worst thing that could happen.

My mind began to race and to consider so many other things. I thought about the tough year Wesley and I had after his dad died; how hard we had been working while trying to go to school; how much I felt like I was carrying us emotionally at times. I remember during that time feeling that I just wanted two things: to be taken care of for a while and to be near my family. Reading that book made me realize that it had taken something terrible to get what I had been wanting, but now I was being taken care of and I was home with my family.

In the moments after this realization, I walked toward my bedroom window to watch the children I could hear playing outside. On the window's mist, I drew a heart and watched it drip into obscurity. I looked at the children, who seemed carefree and I wished them a life that their parents were probably already trying to give them, just as mine had tried to give me. I wished them peace and happiness, but more than that, I wished them the ability to know what they had in their place in life and to appreciate its gifts. Had I not lived my life in that way? Maybe not all of the time. And just before this, maybe not at all. But I made a promise to myself then that I would start. I promised to embrace whatever was coming, and to know that if my will had been, even in part, strong enough to confuse my body into cancer, then my will was definitely strong enough to give my body a way back to health.

The mystery was over, and I decided to no longer question how, but I decided that it was safe to question why. For if I did not search for the answers to why, then I would never find any.

I will get the gallium dye injected into my veins later this afternoon, and then they'll start taking pictures of my insides tomorrow. They'll take pictures for two days this time. I am nervous about getting the results, but I have been in constant prayer since I found out about the test. Dear God, please be with us all.

Wednesday, April 17

On this day, I learned about something that I don't think I could truly define before. On this day, more than any other day, I learned about joy.

As I lay on the table for my gallium scan, remembering

what the one before had looked like months ago, I kept telling myself not to look at the screen. I kept begging myself not to, but I did it anyway.

I had been on the table, laying flat on my back, for nearly fifteen minutes, so I knew that the machine had scanned enough of my body for me to tell if there was any change, enough change, since the last one. The last one—that's all I kept thinking about. I tried to remind myself of how far I had come and what that meant for my body and my spirit. I tried telling myself that no matter what the test showed, I would be healed eventually. But then I started to question what "eventually" meant and if my body could survive six more treatments. All of these thoughts raced through my mind, until finally, I took a deep breath, moved my head carefully so I would not distort the rest of the scan, and then looked over my shoulder to the screen behind me.

And there it was—another picture of my insides. Only I didn't think it was actually a picture of myself. I thought it must have been an example of what a body should look like on the inside and they would later compare mine to that. I looked back again and again, questioning to whom that image on the screen belonged. Could it possibly be me? Could all of the darkness have possibly disappeared and been replaced by the perfection I saw?

Just then, the technician came in the room, and I had to ask him, "On the screen behind me, who is that a picture of?"

He chuckled and answered, "What do you mean? Who do you think that is? It's you up there."

I swallowed hard and paused for a moment. "It's me?" I questioned him further.

"It's you," he answered, and then he left the room.

Tears began to well up in my eyes. I tried to hold them back, but then I wondered why, so I let them fall. I lay there as still as I could and kept turning my head to see the screen.

All I could see was a skeleton, my skeleton, silhouetted in white. It was the most perfect shade of white I had ever seen, and I knew that if there were clouds of white in heaven, then that was the color of white they would be. I turned around again and again, looking at the screen, still questioning if that could possibly be me.

And when I turned for what must have been the hundredth time, I began to sob. In that moment, I felt God telling me, "It's you. You receive it. You've asked for it, you've earned it, now receive it. Receive it." And in that moment, I did. I sobbed as I looked at the screen, finally believing it was my image looking back at me. I cried and I cried, as I lay still, waiting for the machine to stop scanning the rest of me. Briefly, I became fearful that it would find something in my lower body, but I dismissed that thought as fast as it came. I knew I had been healed. And as the tears fell down the sides of my face and dripped down into my ears, I said out loud, "I've received it. Thank you God. I've received it."

Just then, the technician entered with a copy of my old tests. He held them up to the light and said, "I'm no doctor, but it doesn't take a medical degree to see the difference between then and now."

I looked at the old pictures and for the first time, I felt disconnected from the cancer that I saw and that I had felt inside of me for so many months. I knew that the cancer no longer lived inside of me and that I was free of it.

The technician put his hand on my forehead and said quietly, "We'll do this again tomorrow, but you're almost done here. I'm sure there's someplace else you'd rather be." Then he left the room.

Oddly, there really wasn't any other place I'd rather be. I didn't want to leave that moment, because it was a gift. I believed that I had been given a miracle and that part of the experience was to feel the joy—to enjoy the moment.

As I drove home, I spoke out loud to myself, to God, and to whoever else was listening. I spoke of the miracle I had been given; I spoke of the joy my family would get to feel after such a long battle with uncertainty; and I spoke of the gift that I would try to give back for what I had been given.

I had asked Wesley to let me go to this appointment alone, so I could drive there in silence. He respected my wishes and said he would wait for me at home. Wesley was waiting outside for me when I got there. I pulled into the driveway, leaped toward him and hugged him as tightly as I ever had, "We'll keep this quiet until we hear for sure from the doctor, but I didn't see any cancer today. For the first time, I didn't even feel cancer today."

I didn't have to tell him any more than that. Our embrace was long, our tears were large and our hearts were overflowing with joy—pure, perfect joy.

Thursday, April 18

I struggled with myself again today to not look at the screen, fearing that maybe the dye had not penetrated deeply enough to some of the darkened areas yesterday. When I finally did look, I saw something that looked like a different shade of white, but not black at all. My heart began to race. Questions began to pile up inside of my mind. I wondered what I was seeing on the screen and if it was cancer. Was it little enough to allow me to stop the chemo and begin radiation? Had the chemo done its work?

My questions were interrupted by the technician's entrance. I finally decided to just ask him. "What is that area there?"

"That's your sternum," he answered. And once again, he left me to my joy.

I lay on the table for the rest of the scan, but I didn't even bother to look at the screen again, because I already knew. All I wanted was to finish, go home, call the doctor and tell the rest of my family.

Wesley insisted on being with me for today's gallium scan and was in the waiting room when I finished. He said, "Well?"

"All clear!" I answered. We cried as we did the day before. Then, I tried to call Dr. Verma when we got home.

Kim said he would be out of the office until Monday, so he would call me with the results when he returned. I hung up the phone knowing that I was not going to wait until Monday for his call or confirmation of what I already knew. I had met the radiologist who was handling my tests when I went the first day for the injection of the gallium dye, so I decided to call him myself. Having cancer had taught me many things, one of which was to follow my own instincts and be assertive when dealing with doctors and other health care workers. And assertive I was.

I called and asked to speak with Dr. Lee. He came to the phone immediately. I asked him for the results, and he said that he would review them and call me back.

I waited only fifteen minutes, when the phone rang. It was Dr. Lee.

"Lisa, I have looked over all of your scans, and I don't see any cancer. It's as if it has all disappeared. There isn't a trace of it anywhere." he explained.

"Not anywhere?" I asked.

"Not anywhere," he answered.

I sat there for a brief second and decided to ask the one question that had been on my mind. I felt it would completely put me at ease to have it answered. "How do you know the dye went in properly? What if that's why nothing is showing up?"

"I can see the dye all throughout your body. In your spleen, in your liver, but it's not cancer. Lisa, I cannot see any cancer," he reassured me.

I thanked him and hung up the phone. Wesley already knew the answer to my question and the answer to our prayers.

"Call your parents," he told me.

When I did, the desk clerk at the hotel said they weren't in their room. "Okay, then will you write down this message?" I asked her.

"Sure, what is it?"

"Just say that Lisa called and write 'It's all gone!'" I told her.

"It's all gone?" she questioned me, not knowing what that meant.

"They'll know what it means," I said.

She said she'd give them the message, then said good-bye.

I tried to call everyone who had been waiting for the results along with us, but it was still early in the day, so everyone was at work or at school. We left messages all over town, and then decided to celebrate.

We went to dinner, to the park, and just drove around laughing and smiling—two things we hadn't done much of in months. And when we returned home, the answering machine was full of messages. *Everyone* had called us back. My Aunt Jeri was the first. She was crying and the kids and my Grandma Shaw were cheering in the background. She finally said she had to hang up, because it was so emotional for them.

Darla and my Aunt Joyce called next. They kept saying how happy they were for us and how proud they were of me for being so strong throughout the whole thing.

Bev called while we were listening to the messages. She was crying and thanking God over and over again.

My brother and Heather had called, too. He said, "Oh,

Lisa, my sister, you're going to be okay!"

I hadn't reached my Grandma Smith, my mom's mom, when I called the others earlier, so I tried calling her again.

"Grandma, I have good news," I told her when she answered the phone.

"What, baby?" she asked.

"I don't have cancer anymore! My test was all clear!"

"Oh, baby!" she was crying. "Oh I'm so glad you don't have to have those treatments anymore! Oh, baby!" she kept crying and that made me cry even more, because I have never heard my grandma cry. She's one of the strongest women I have ever known, and to hear her cry tears of joy, made me realize how torturous this, too, had been for her.

While I was talking to my grandma, my parents called on the other line. I didn't even get to say hello, I could already hear them on the other line. They were sharing the phone receiver. They were crying, "We love you, Lisa! Oh, God, we love you! No more cancer! Wow!" they cried.

"Isn't it great!" I said.

"Oh, it's more than great! I told you, honey," my dad said.

"I know Dad! You were right," I said as Wesley and I also shared the phone receiver and even more tears of joy.

When we were done talking to everyone, we just stood looking at each other. It was almost as if we didn't know what to do with ourselves. These were new people looking at each other. Renewed people. I was bald, had lost more than twenty-five pounds, my clothes hung on me, and my face was pale with dark circles under my eyes, but I had never felt more alive. Wesley took my hand and led me to our bedroom, making the perfect ending to a perfect day.

On this day, for the first time since December 26, I feel like I have some of what I lost back—some of what made me who I was before the whole thing fell apart and the cancer entered my life. The doctors would say that the test was good news and there was still more work to do, but I choose to rest and rally in the knowledge that my body has begun to heal and my spirit feels free. I can begin to trust in my body again, because for so very long I did not.

I see so much more than I did before. And even though I feel I got an old part of myself back with the good news of no cancer in the sight of the gallium, I won't be the same person I was before this experience. I don't want to be. That would mean all of this happened for no reason at all—nothing learned, nothing gained.

I have gained some things and I have lost some things, and I am truly okay with that. I can't say that I am ready to shout it from a rooftop, but I'm ready to smile more than I did before and trust that what we did worked.

I can't continue to write, because all I want to do right now is listen to music, be with Wesley and enjoy the rest of the night and the peace this day has brought me. I have thanked God. I have received it, and I am finally, after years of knowing him, learning about the power of prayer and his absolute love for me. I thank Wesley, my parents and the rest of my family for taking such good care of me. Thank God, no more cancer!

Twelve

Thursday, April 25

"It's kind of scary," I told the doctor.

"What is?" Dr. Bobba asked.

"The darkness, the glow of the bulbs shining down on me," I explained.

"Am *I* scaring you?"

"No, it's not you. It's all of it," I answered.

"We'll be finished shortly. Then, we won't have to do this again," he said.

I had been under the small lights for several minutes. Chemotherapy ended. Radiation was beginning.

I had met Dr. Bobba, my radiology oncologist once before when he filled in for Dr. Verma during my doctor visit after the gallium scan. Earlier this morning, he explained the risks of radiation and chemotherapy combined, which were what Dr. Verma had explained to me before I started chemotherapy. The one risk I had not considered or been told about yet was the risk of breast cancer from having radiation to my chest. He explained that they would be molding three-inch-thick lead plates that would rest on the radiation machine and would shield my lungs from the beams of light that were supposed to be instrumental for my cure.

Dr. Bobba also had a large marker and wrote all over my chest with it. I didn't know what the measurements were for, exactly, but he assured me that the ink would easily wash off. They took X-rays of my chest to figure out exactly where to place the lead shields. Then, they marked my chest in three spots with a small dot tattoo, so they would not have to measure the area each time, and so there would be a permanent record of where I had been treated. I didn't like the idea of having tattoo marks on my chest, no matter how small, but I remained compliant in the choices I had made. The technicians were very nice and talked me through the entire procedure. They told me that many patients have said that, compared to chemotherapy, radiation is a walk in the park. Radiation doesn't usually cause any problems with white or red blood cell counts, so I will no longer have to give myself shots. Dr. Bobba also said I would experience fatigue and possibly some irritation on my skin and in my throat, but that if I kept my chest area moist after the treatments, I might not experience the chapping at all.

I was still thinking about the radiation and my risk for breast cancer. I kept thinking about the movies I had seen that dealt with radiation poisoning and it scared me. The doctor assured me that the treatments were a very controlled process and that they had come a long way in treating Hodgkin's disease and administering radiation for those treatments. Dr. Bobba said that years ago they used to over-radiate because they wanted to make sure they were killing the cancer, but they didn't know then that it didn't require so much treatment. I had heard that many of the patients who were treated more than fifteen or twenty years ago never had a recurrence of Hodgkin's, but they did have heart trouble and hardened arteries from too much radiation.

The whole thing made me uneasy, but I wasn't going to stop now. I had asked Mary about the risks from radiation and told her I had considered not even having the radiation treatments since the gallium was already clear.

"I think that would be a mistake, because the radiation makes sure that all of the little cancer cells, if any, that cannot be seen in a test are killed. If even one cell is left it can grow and multiply and you'll have to go through this all over again," she said. "Don't stop now; you're almost done."

In the beginning, I had told Mary that I didn't want to hear about any other patients who's had Hodgkin's, because I was afraid to hear about all of them who'd died. She agreed not to speak about them. During our conversation about radiation, however, I finally asked her how many of her patients had died.

"In all of the twenty-one years I have been an oncology nurse, I have only known one of my patients to die of this disease. She was a drug addict who stopped showing up for her radiation treatments and didn't finish treatment and never returned for follow-up to monitor her progress. The cancer came back, and it was months before she returned for treatment. By then, it was too late," she explained.

I wondered, when she told me of only one person dying of Hodgkin's in all of her years of treating it, she never told me that before. I always figured she knew several people who had died of it. When I mentioned it to Wesley he said, "She never said anything about anyone else because you asked her not to."

He was right. That's one of the many things that I loved about Mary. No matter what she thought, she left me in control of my treatment and my disease. She was there to help in any way possible, but the decisions were left up to me.

At my appointment with Dr. Verma on Tuesday, I got confirmation from him that I was, in fact, done with chemotherapy.

He discussed it with me and told me that in his opinion, the chemotherapy had done its work and it was time to move forward. Strangely, it seemed that the subject was up for discussion. I had figured he would tell me what to do next, but I appreciated him including me in the process of choosing what would be best. After all, it is my body and my cancer we are discussing.

I went to see Mary after that appointment with Dr. Verma. I showed up with a big smile on my face and I wasn't dressed in my usual sweats and sweatshirt for treatment. I started wearing regular clothes after the second treatment because the itching stopped.

She took one look at me and said, "You're done with chemo, aren't you?"

"The gallium was perfectly clear. Not a spot of cancer to be seen!" I explained.

She hugged me and got teary-eyed. Her sincere joy was so apparent. I'd miss her, but I promised to visit her again. As much as I would miss her, I knew that part of my journey was complete and the only place to go from there was forward.

Before I begin radiation, I have to repeat the lung test to make sure there was no permanent damage caused by the chemotherapy. The tests are not bothering me as much as they did when all of this began. The fear of the unknown has diminished. I feel stronger and more in control of the outcome now. Knowing that I am nearing the end of treatment entirely has enabled me to look into the future. Before the clear gallium, I was afraid to look too far ahead, because all I could see was the struggle I faced. Now I see the possibility of life, the likelihood of survival.

I also have much to look forward to in the month ahead. I can see that radiation may become secondary to the events that are planned. My cousin Corinee, her husband James and her daughter Kayla will be here next weekend. My brother will be here soon after that. My best friend since eighth grade, Tracy, will be here in two weeks. She and I had drifted apart in recent years, and she's the first to admit that much of our distance has been her fault. I have tried, over the years, to bridge the gap that our distance in miles created, but it wasn't until I called her to say I had cancer that we both realized the value of our friendship. None of that matters now. What does matter is that I have my best friend back, and I know that we will both work harder to be in touch and share in each other's lives. I've missed her, and I consider our renewed friendship one of the blessings I have discovered along this journey. Tracy will be coming from Los Angeles, and I can't wait to see her.

I am equally excited about seeing my brother for the first time since this began. I feel a new sense of oneness with him. I feel a sense of acceptance that we did not have before, and I truly believe that whatever has caused conflict in our relationship before this came to our lives has been replaced by a requited love that neither of us believed was possible before. I sent him the journal entry I wrote after reading the book about creative visualization he sent. He and Heather replied with a beautiful card and wrote how much they admired me for the way I was handling this misfortune. Vance wrote: "I am so proud of my sister and her knowledge. You're showing all who are lucky to be close to you what is important to you and how healthy spiritually and physically you've become."

I love Vance for many things that I didn't know about him before I faced this battle. More than any of those newfound things, I love him for telling me he loves me every time we speak now. The days of childhood spent distancing ourselves from one another are only a reminder of the mistakes we made all of those years ago. Mistakes I truly believe we will never repeat.

The month ahead will bring some uncertainty. But unlike

the months before, a balance exists now. I dredged through the bad, because I was faithful that the good would eventually come. It is here now. It is waiting for me and will only remain if I allow it. I want nothing more than for the days ahead to bring forth the peace we all deserve.

We have begun to plan my got-well party. I made the guest list and am inviting everyone who sent a card and those who called to lend good wishes. I keep a picture of what I expect from that day in my thoughts, and I know the day is not far off. We now deem it possible and welcome its arrival. It is set for June 8. And on that day, we will all breathe a sigh of relief from the light that will be found at the end of our tunnel. And maybe, if we allow it, the darkness will be gone forever.

Wednesday, May 1

I started radiation today. It really was easy. I received thirty seconds of radiation on each side, my back and my chest. With the tiny tattoo marks on my chest, Matt, one of the technicians, knows exactly where to place the lead shields and wastes little time getting things ready.

Wesley met me there for treatment after playing golf with my dad. He was a little late getting there, but I didn't even mind. It was as simple as Matt had promised. Wesley was nervous about being late, but I reassured him that not only did I not mind, but he also didn't need to accompany me to the rest of my treatments. For some reason, I felt like this was something I could do on my own. And since I could, I wanted to.

Without the side effects of chemotherapy, I feel like a new person. I have been walking on the golf course in the evenings, and Wesley and I have continued playing tennis. I have heard that radiation is cumulative and causes fatigue after a while, but I can handle that. I am just tired of being sick and tired.

Tuesday, May 7

Corinee, James and Kayla were here over the weekend. It was good to see them. We were able to shop and have lunch on Saturday, because I have been feeling pretty good. I had planned to go with the family out on my parents' boat on Sunday, but I was too tired. I think the week's radiation caught up with me, but I have no complaints. They left on Sunday afternoon and will hopefully be back in June for the party.

I had blood work done this morning. Dr. Bobba and Dr. Verma wanted to make sure that my blood counts had regulated after completing chemotherapy. My counts are stable and are nearing the proper range.

I hadn't been to the lab in a while. The ladies were glad to see I am doing so well. They said they started to get worried when I didn't show up for a few weeks.

The week has actually been rather uneventful. I keep my chest area moist with lotion after treatment and, so far, haven't experienced any irritation or peeling. I do not have any soreness in my throat or difficulty swallowing. It seems the physical effects of chemotherapy have already diminished. I no longer have to spend every day wondering what could go wrong with my body. I no longer look for signs of serious complications. I am able to just live from day to day, going in for my treatments at 11:00 A.M. each day and waiting for it all to be over.

Tracy will be here on Friday.

Monday, May 13

When I first saw Tracy, it felt like coming home after a long trip to find the most comfortable place to rest. I hadn't seen her in three years, but it was as if we had never been apart. We shopped, she bought me lunch, and we even got to see a movie. Those are the things we always did when we lived near each other, and in between, we talked about everything. Some things never change, and I found myself sitting at a restaurant bar, waiting for a table, watching all of the men watch her. She's never married, was engaged once, but is still single and likes it that way. I know that she noticed the men around us. It was not a confidence booster for me, to say the least, because I was sitting there with next-to-no hair and what curves of desire I did have left with the last ten pounds I'd lost.

While Tracy was here, I convinced her to try something new with her hair. As pretty as it was, she'd been wearing it long and curly for many years and she could stand a change. She agreed.

We went to her aunt's salon. Tracy was getting her hair cut in layers and loving it, while I sat in the chair next to her and noticed a few changes of my own.

"Oh my," I said, as I walked closer to the mirror.

"What is it? What's the matter?" Tracy asked.

"It's my eyebrows. I have none," I answered.

"What do you mean? You have eyebrows," she replied.

"Barely. I guess I hadn't noticed, because I rarely put makeup on these days," I said, still looking closely in the mirror at my face. "This is really weird."

Tracy asked her aunt to stop cutting and walked over to me. "Are you okay?" she asked.

I looked surprised by her question, but I understood its origination. She thought that losing my eyebrows upset me. It didn't.

"Oh Trac. My eyebrows—that's nothing. It's all going to be over soon. They'll come back, and so will the rest of me," I said. More for her than for myself, I gave her a hug. Tears welled up in her eyes. "Are *you* okay?" I asked her.

"Yeah. I'm just marveling at my brave friend," she answered.

Tracy left this morning. I miss her already.

Thursday, May 16

I am tired all of the time. I sleep about twelve hours during the night and then nap again for a few hours during the day. Toward the beginning of the week I feel fine, but then the cumulative effects of the radiation tire me by the week's end. Being tired isn't difficult, because I just sleep when I need to, but I can feel my patience wearing thin each day. My dad has been home this week, and his constant positive attitude finally pushed me over the edge.

We were sitting in the kitchen talking about the treatments when it began. I always knew that the worst thing that could be said in our house growing up was "I can't," but I thought that my dad would let this one go given the circumstances.

"The worst part right now is that I can't take a deep breath; it hurts," I told them.

"Well, don't say 'I can't,'" my dad said.

As soon as he said those words, I felt myself boiling over inside. I wanted to run out of the house screaming. I wanted to kick something. I wanted to pull what was left of my hair out. I could do none of these things. I just sat there and began my rebuttal.

"Dad! This isn't me telling you that I can't hit the ball or that I can't work a math problem. This is so much bigger than that. You have no idea!"

"But maybe if you don't think about what you can't do and think about what you can do, then you will feel better," he said.

"Dad! You don't understand. This is not about my will; it's about what is physically wrong with me. I'm taxed! Don't you get it?" I yelled.

"Lisa, your dad is just trying to help," my mom said in his defense.

"Well, he's not," I yelled. "He's not helping!" I stormed out of the room and into my bedroom where Wesley was reading a magazine. They asked me to come back to the kitchen, but I ignored them and shut the door and locked it. I was furious!

"Are you listening to this?" I asked Wesley.

"I'm not getting involved," he said.

"But are you listening to this?" I asked him again.

Just then, I heard the doorknob jiggle. "Lisa, unlock this door," my mom said.

"She locked the door?" I heard my dad ask her.

"No, just leave me alone. I don't want to talk anymore. The conversation is over!" I exclaimed.

"This isn't fair, Lisa. You're not being fair," my mom said.

"Well, in case you haven't noticed, life just isn't fair sometimes," and as soon as the words left my mouth I saw Wesley look at me in contempt.

"That was uncalled for," he said quietly.

"Yeah, well, I thought you were staying out of this!" I snapped back at him.

Then I was trapped. I wasn't getting what I wanted from Wesley, my parents were still waiting on the other side of the door for me, and I was as far from an apology as I had ever been in my life. Were they really expecting an apology?

I opened the door and walked between my parents. "I'm leaving," I told them.

"Where are you going?" my dad asked.

"Just anywhere. Somewhere!" I shouted as I walked down the hallway. As I walked farther away from them and toward the kitchen to find my car keys, I knew I had crossed a very fine line. I knew that I was taking my anger out on them and I was being, as my mother said, unfair. But I felt like I had backed myself into a corner, and I didn't want to back down. I knew that there were things I was feeling and saying that were going against what all of us had worked toward in our union against the cancer, but I was just too mad to explain any of it to them. Rather than walking out the door, I sat back down at the kitchen table. I would give it one more try.

"What is going on with you, Lisa?" my dad asked. "I have tried telling you before that I can't be the one who cries with you about this. I can't be the one you talk with about the toll it all has taken on you. That's not my role here."

"I know it isn't. I've heard you every time you have explained it. But you just don't get it. Nobody seems to get it!" I said firmly.

"Don't get what? That you don't feel well? That you are tired of the treatments and they are wearing you down?" my dad asked.

"No Dad! It's none of those things!" I shouted.

"Then what is it?" he pressed further. "What is it!"

"I'm angry!" I cried. "I'm angry! For the first time since all of this began I haven't had to think about the effects that treatment is having on my body. So now what? Now all of these things go through my mind and all I can do is wonder what will become of me. When all of this is done and the treatments do their job, what will become of what is left of me? Will there be anything left of me? How do I go through the rest of my life and live with what went on here? How do I ever forget and learn to live with it?"

I was holding my face in my hands, and I was sobbing. I looked up to see that my parents were also crying. Finally, for the first time since I was diagnosed, my dad was crying. They both walked toward me, and without saying a word, they held my weeping face in their hands. I was the first to speak again.

"And in the end, I'm still the one who had cancer. I'll always be the one who had cancer," I cried.

"Don't you know that every single day we wish it were us that got sick instead of you? Don't you know that your mother and I cried and begged God to spare your life and take ours instead? We're your parents, Lisa. We just keep asking ourselves how we survived watching you struggle," my dad explained.

"But for months I have been dealing with the physical effects of cancer. And now, after thinking I was so strong, I have realized that I haven't even begun to deal with my mind. I haven't begun to deal with what this has done to my heart, my spirit, the part of me that has to find a way to live with the cancer even after it's gone," I said to them.

"But we just can't be anything but happy to know that our daughter will survive. And so now you have won the battle, Lisa. It's almost over," my mother explained.

"But that's just it. That's what you don't get," I said quietly. "I'm afraid the battle may have just begun."

Friday, May 17

When I am feeling weak, God sends me a gift to help me realize that redemption is not far off. I will, one day, be able to retrieve the peace of mind I so desire. On this day, he sent me the gift of my brother. Vance arrived today.

I heard them pull into the driveway, so I met them at the door. I had my hat on, so I would not shock them with what little hair I had left. I wanted Vance to see me in the best possible light.

I opened the door and saw Vance running toward the door. Before Heather reached the front porch, Vance and I had embraced.

"Oh, my sister. My sister!" Vance said as he released his embrace to look at me. "You don't look bad at all. It looks like you have a lot of hair under that hat."

"Well, I don't. But that's okay. It's so good to see you," I said as a few tears fell from my eyes.

By then, Heather and Wesley had both reached the door, and while we all exchanged hugs, I felt good again and hoped that the little things along the way would restore my desire to seek what would heal my aching spirit.

Sunday, May 19

It seemed like they left as quickly as they arrived. At least I know they will be back for the party next month. We had a great time with them. My brother and Heather were very generous, taking us to dinner and renting movies for all of us to watch. They took us to eat sushi. Wesley and I had never eaten it before, and neither one of us liked it very much. I couldn't eat any raw seafood or fish, so I was limited. But it was fun to try something new.

We didn't talk much about the cancer; not because we were avoiding the subject but because we have talked about it numerous times over the phone, and it seemed like it was secondary to the time we were able to spend together. It felt freeing, in a way, to have our weekend be about something more than what has been the focus of our lives for so many months now.

I know that I will miss Vance in the time we spend apart now. For years, we have lived at a great distance from one another, but our separation had little impact on our lives. We have been glad to see each other in the years of our adulthood, but I think now it will mean something different to spend time together.

While they were here, Heather and I talked about Vance's reaction to my illness. Until then, I never really considered what that phone call must have been like for him. I knew it made my father cry. I asked her how Vance took the news.

"We had company that day, so we were visiting with them when the phone rang. Vance answered," she explained. "I wasn't paying much attention to his end of the conversation at first, but when he started to cry out loud I stopped talking with our friends to find out what had him so upset."

"Vance cried?" I asked.

"Yeah, he cried. I heard him say to your dad, 'She has cancer? What do you mean she has cancer? Is she going to die?' Then, he looked at me and said, 'It's Lisa, she's sick.'"

"I had no idea he took it so hard," I said to her. It didn't make me feel good to hear these things, but it did make me realize a bit more about his love for me.

I thought a lot about what Heather and I talked about. I thought about how it must've been for my brother to be so far away from us while I went through the early stages of the diagnosis and then chemotherapy. I told my mom what Heather told me and she said that the last time she and Vance spoke he said, "I never knew that I loved my sister until now. Now I can say I love her." My heart just melted when she told me. It made me wish he were still here so I could give him another hug or tell him I loved him again, but I know that our time together these past few days was rich in our expressing our love for one another.

Since I was diagnosed with cancer, I have tried to be conscious of the events that transpire each day. I want to live each day of this in a way that will not leave me with any regrets. That's why I say what I need to say to the people I love and I do the things that need to be done to help me survive. And for this, I know that Vance and I spent a perfect time together, and I have no regrets and nothing more needed to be said. I love him. He knows that now. And he loves me. As I become aware of the blessings that have come to my life because of this experience, I count this simple yet momentous realization among the most endearing.

Wednesday, May 22

While I was at radiation today, Matt kept asking me if I was feeling all right. I felt tired and run down. He asked Dr. Bobba to order some blood work. It scares me to ponder what could be wrong. I just keep waiting for someone to call and tell me everything is okay. Lately, I feel like my heart has been skipping a beat here and there, but it does not quite feel like a palpitation. I don't know what is causing it, but I'll feel better once I know what my blood results are.

I went to see Dr. McCabe again on Monday. He wanted to see how I was holding up through radiation. Bev went with me. She told me afterward that she doesn't like him. He scares her with his brutal honesty. To me, it's a comfort, because I always know he is telling the truth. I asked him questions, and he gave me answers.

I still didn't understand what the fifteen-year survival rate meant for Hodgkin's patients. I wanted him to explain it to me.

"So this fifteen-year survival rate, what does that mean? Does it mean that I am going to go through all of this and then die when I'm forty-nine years old instead of twenty-four?" I asked Dr. McCabe.

"No, what that means is that at the end of fifteen years, 85 percent of the people who had Hodgkin's disease are still alive."

"So that has nothing to do with what could happen to me then?" I pressed further.

"It just means that most people who recover from this go on to live healthy, normal, productive lives," he answered.

The main question I wanted answered clearly was how long I should wait to have children. I told him my menstrual cycle was normal throughout treatment.

"That's a good sign," he said.

"So how long should I wait to have kids? Should I wait until the five-year survival mark when they tell me I'm cured?"

"Why would you want to do that?" he asked.

"I don't *want* to do that. I'm just wondering if I *should* do that," I said.

"Look at it this way: You could go through this treatment, and then two years later this stuff could come back in some wicked, spooky form and you'd die," he explained. "But if you had a baby, you'd have something of yourself to leave behind. Something that said you were here. Your parents would be grandparents. Besides, you could leave here today and get hit by a bus. Then what?"

"So I don't have to be cured to get pregnant?" I asked.

"You can't live your life waiting to be cured of this. You need to find a new way to live so you can deal with what has happened to you, but don't put your life on hold because of it," he said.

When I got home from seeing Dr. McCabe, I took a shower. The things he said kept running through my mind, and all I could think about was the worst-case scenario he gave me, and it wasn't the one about getting hit by a bus. While I thought these horrific thoughts, I began compulsively checking for lumps all over my body. I started thinking about the man I heard about who went through chemotherapy and had no signs of cancer, then after radiation they did one more scan to be sure and it was back, only this time it was everywhere, even in his legs. I knew that this man went through more treatment and got well and is alive today, but I just kept thinking about him and wondering if the same could happen to me. I kept thinking about the risks that I was warned about—leukemia, second tumors and infertility. All of these things raced recklessly through my mind, until suddenly, it stopped. My mind was silent, and as I reached for the shampoo to wash what was left of my hair, it was like a light went on to show me how out of control I was. Amazingly, something brought me out of that raging fear and told me not to worry. I'm worrying about cancers that I will probably never get, and even if I did, doctors could have a cure for them when my fifteen-year survival time was up. As harsh as some of what he said seemed even to me, I knew he was speaking the truth. I knew I needed to find a new way to live each day, so I wouldn't spend the rest of my life fearing what could happen to me. I guess that's what had me so upset with my parents the other day. Now that the treatment for my body is coming to an end, it's time to start dealing with the things that run through my mind every day. It's time to start thinking about something other than cancer when I wake up in the morning and when I go to bed each night. How long it will take to gain some kind of control over these thoughts, I do not know. But I must begin to try.

4:54 P.M.—Dr. Bobba just called. I could hear Wesley talking to him. I was in my room getting very nervous about the blood results. Wesley tried calming me down, but it didn't work. When the phone rang, I told him to answer it. I couldn't take any bad news.

"Everything is fine," he told me when he entered our bedroom.

"What do you mean? The blood work came back okay?" I asked.

"All of your counts are in normal range. Dr. Bobba said it's to be expected that you are getting so tired now that you are nearing the end of this regimen," Wesley explained.

"Did you tell him about my heart?"

"Yeah. He said that if it continues or worsens then you should go see Dr. Verma about it," he said.

"So, I'm fine," I said, almost as a question, rather than a statement.

"You're fine," Wesley said as he kissed me on the lips. "Do you want to go out for dinner?"

"Yeah, I do," I answered.

I don't know why I was shocked by the news of everything being okay. I guess I'll have to start getting used to things going better for me. After months of nothing but trials and tribulations, it's hard for me to imagine that my life might actually be spared of this ever happening again. I'll have to start thinking in those terms, otherwise, what would be the point of this gift of life if I were unable to appreciate it.

I started to shave what was left of my hair yesterday. I've lost most of it, but because I had such thick hair, whatever is left was extra and probably won't fall out. It stopped falling out a few days ago. That's why I wanted to shave my head, so I could start fresh. It made everyone in the house nervous. However it made me feel, I only managed to shave the very top, then I got scared and stopped. Even that doesn't really matter, because I always wear one of the hats my mom sewed me. It's obvious to strangers that I'm a young woman with cancer. I still get the pity looks.

Sunday, May 26

I was sitting at the table this morning eating breakfast when my mom started looking closely at my head. I asked her what she was looking at.

"I can see little hairs all over your head, just a shadow of dark hair coming in," she said.

"You mean new hair? You mean it's growing back?" I asked her as I walked toward the mirror in the living room. She was right. My hair was growing back, and it was very dark. "So let's shave the old stuff off! Let's start anew today!" I exclaimed.

"Are you sure you want to do that?" my mom asked.

"Yeah, it's not like I can wear a hat for the next year while I wait for the new hair to catch up with what's left. You want to help me Wesley?"

"I don't think I can," he said. "It would make me too nervous," he answered.

"How about you, Mom?"

"I don't really want to either. Why don't you go ask your dad to do it?" she suggested.

I headed for the back door, where I found him sitting on the deck outside.

"Come on, Dad. I've got new hair growing in. You're going to help me shave the old stuff off," I told him.

"Oh, I don't know about that, Lisa. I don't know," he hesitated.

"Come on, Dad. You're the tough guy. Let's get this done," I persuaded him as I pulled him out of his chair.

"Are you sure you want to do this?" my dad asked as we headed for the bathroom.

"Positive," I answered.

We used the clippers that were under the sink and set them on the longest setting of one-fourth inch. As the hair began to fall from my head and onto the floor, I felt that each strand of hair represented the weight that was being lifted from my shoulders. For months, I'd felt like I had the weight of the world riding on my back. No matter where I was or what I was doing, there was a burden that could not be lifted. The agony had been relentless throughout, and only during very rare moments did I actually forget that I had cancer. I'd wake up in the morning and for a brief second, I might not be aware of the cancer, and then it would come to me in a wave of grief. But while my dad shaved my head, and I began to see the baldness underneath the straggly hair that had been left behind after months of chemotherapy, something inside of me rejoiced. Something inside of me said that this was only the beginning of good things to come. And just like when I was laying on the gallium scan table looking at the clear picture of a cancer-free body, I allowed a breath of joy to filter into the moment, and I rejoiced for yet another gift I was being given. And for my dad, I think he may have finally found his place in all of this. I needed him today and he was there for me. He, at first, didn't want to be the one to do it, but then I think he must have wondered who else could? Just my dad, that's who. Just my dad.

Tuesday, May 28

When Wesley woke me up this morning, I felt like it was the last day of school and summer was about to begin.

"Lisa, it's time to get up," he said as he lay next to me. "This is it. It's your last day."

I was sound asleep when he entered the room, still feeling tired from the radiation treatments, but I felt amazingly well knowing that it was all about to end. I smiled as I rolled over to greet him and the day.

"Your mom gave me some money to take you to lunch after your treatment is over. She wants us to enjoy ourselves and celebrate. So get up, let's get going," he said as he kissed me and walked toward the door.

I got up from my bed and walked toward the window. The same three kids I'd been watching play outside all winter and spring were there again. I watched them for a moment and thought about all of the times I played on the same street as a child. I thought about how lucky I always felt in my family and amongst our close friends, because there were so many special people in our lives, and I wondered if everyone had such a close knit of family and friends. Ironically, on this day, I felt lucky again. I felt like I was doing something so big that anything else would pale in comparison.

On the way out the door for treatment, I picked up three note cards and put them in my bag.

"What are those?" Wesley asked.

"I wrote Dr. Bobba, Matt and Maureen, the other technician, thank-you cards. I just wanted them to know what their help has meant to me. I may never see them again. It only seems right that I thank them for helping save my life," I explained.

"I'm sure they'll appreciate it," Wesley said as he put his hand on the middle of my back and led me out the front door. As he did, I thought about all of the times before that he had taken me to appointments and treatments; rubbed my arms when they hurt; given me the shots when I couldn't give them to myself; taken care of me when I was sick; how every single time I needed him during the past months he had been there without fail or question.

"Wesley, wait a minute," I said as I stopped him in front of the car.

"What's the matter? Did you forget something?" he asked.

"No, it's not that," I answered.

"What is it?" he asked. "Are you okay?"

My eyes filled with tears. "It's you. *You* saved my life. You saved my life every single day."

He reached for my hand, and then wiped the tears from my face.

"You saved me, too," he said. And after a long embrace, we got into the car and drove to the last treatment of cancer we would ever have to endure.

When the treatment was over, we said our good-byes to each of the staff, and I gave them their cards of thanks. They said people don't usually do that, and I said, "Well, maybe they should."

When we got into the car, I asked Wesley where he was taking me. He said he'd made a reservation at a small restaurant nearby. It was right across the street.

When we entered the restaurant, the hostess said she'd been expecting us. "Right this way," she said.

We followed her into a room in the back, where there was a large table with people surrounding it. After a few moments, I realized that all of the people sitting at the table were there for me: my mom and dad, both of my grandmas, and my Aunt Jeri. I was so surprised that I could barely speak. There were flowers and balloons everywhere.

"What's going on?" I asked my parents.

"We just thought we'd have an end-of-treatment party with your chemo group before the big party next Saturday," my mom answered. "Bev can't make it because of her knee surgery and Darla is on the way."

"I can't believe you guys did this! This is great! I had no idea!" I exclaimed.

"Didn't you see their cars parked outside?" Wesley asked.

"No, I didn't even notice," I said as I made my way to the seat open next to my mom. There was a gift wrapped for Mary. "Are we going over to the hospital to take this to Mary after lunch?" I asked my mom. She didn't answer me.

"Is Mary coming?" I asked with excitement.

"Yes!" my mom said.

"Did you get her those pearl earrings we saw last week?" I asked.

"Yes, they're beautiful. I hope she likes them."

I sat down at the table and looked around at everyone looking at me in excitement. Wesley pushed my chair in and kissed me on the top of my head. I still wore a hat even though my hair was starting to grow back.

Everyone started talking about how hard it was to keep the lunch a secret, because they were afraid I'd see the cars or that Spencer would tell me at his birthday party last week. It worked out perfectly. I was completely surprised. I had wondered, however, why my dad was still in town on a Tuesday.

Mary arrived within a few minutes. My mom asked her to sit next to me. I hadn't seen her since I finished chemotherapy. I'd missed her.

"Oh you look so wonderful! What a cute hat!" Mary said.

"Yeah look at what we did," I said as I pulled off my hat. "My dad shaved it for me!"

"It looks great. You have a beautiful face and can pull off this look," she said.

"She has a perfectly shaped head, doesn't she?" Wesley added. "I was nervous to see her without hair, but now I think she looks beautiful."

For the rest of the lunch, we all sat and talked about all kinds of things. We talked about the weather; what Wesley and I had been doing with our days since I was feeling better; how much we were looking forward to the got-well party. We talked about everything but cancer. The word, the subject, nor the thought ever came up. It was the beginning of a week-long celebration of what had ended and what was ahead. I felt very loved sitting there amongst the people who had been instrumental in my recovery and it was a day I would never forget.

Sunday, June 2

Yesterday was my Grandma Shaw's seventy-fifth birthday. The whole family was there to celebrate. We threw her a surprise party. All of her kids took her to dinner, but they didn't plan on her wanting to stay and dance the night away. All of the grandchildren were waiting for them to arrive. They were two hours late, because they couldn't get my grandma to leave and they didn't want to tell her about us waiting for her or about the party. They eventually showed up for the party, and she was very surprised and happy to see all of the family together.

Since my grandpa's death more than three years ago, the family has gone its separate ways. When he was diagnosed with cancer, he came up with the idea to have a family dinner every month. He let each of his children take turns choosing the restaurant. It started out just being the immediate family, and then it expanded to the extended family and their children. It became very important to all of us and proved to make us closer in the months before he died. I think that by the time he died a year and a half after he was diagnosed, we were all so saddened by his death that we wanted to retreat from everything that represented the pain we suffered watching him die.

I think that's part of the reason why we were all focusing on a gala celebration for when my treatment ended. With my grandpa's experience, cancer meant death because he never opted for treatment of any kind. He knew that in his circumstances treatment would not prolong his life but take away from its quality. Every story we heard when he was diagnosed was about someone who'd died of cancer, because that is what we were going through at the time. It wasn't until I was diagnosed with cancer that we discovered how many people actually survived. Treatments were working, patients were complying with their doctor's regimens of choice, and people were living. It was the most important discovery, in the beginning, to know that cancer was not a death sentence. For some, it had little impact on their life, depending on the treatment they received. And for others, no matter how difficult the regimen of treatment they received, they still survived and found their way back to good health.

I think patients remaining compliant during the treatment process is also among the most important things to be done that can lead to a full recovery. Maureen said that she only knew two people who had died of Hodgkin's and both of them quit treatment part way through when they started feeling better and didn't return for follow-up. I know that will never be me, no matter how hard it gets to make myself go to a hospital and have another test that will search my body for cancer. I will always take that responsibility very seriously.

I am already beginning to understand the fear I will have to learn to live with. I will have to find a way to rise above it. I remember I called my friend Tami's mom Wanda when I first found out about my cancer. She'd had breast cancer four years before, and when I first spoke with her she told me, "Your life will never be the same. You won't be the same person anymore." I wanted to immediately hang up the phone, because I thought I sensed fear in her voice. I now realize what she meant. It doesn't have to be a life of fear, but I can't change how it has changed me. Once that part of yourself is lost, you can't get it back.

Many of my waking moments are spent in fear of the unknown. I still wonder what my future holds, but what I know I must learn to do is get up every day and find a way to deal with what has happened. As difficult as it has been, this part of it is coming to an end and now I need to move on with my life. Sometimes I think the hardest work is ahead of me, so for now I choose to spend these coming days in celebration and peace. We all must give thanks that what was endured is coming to an end.

It's during these times that the others are free to look at me in a way that no longer resembles pity or fear. They look at me as they look at each other, and—remarkably—the rest has fallen away.

I look at each of them differently also. I look at them like the angels they are. They are the people who helped save my life and, in between the treatments and the sickness and the emotionally taxing pain I suffered, were there to get me to the next day with a little hope and a lot of love. What else is there, I wonder? What could be more important than that?

I reflect on my life, and I can almost see what there was before this. There was good before, and I like to believe there will also be good after. Life is a cycle, and I think that coming out of this darkness will enable me to see what my true purpose is. Why did all of this happen to me? I no longer ask that question because I am angry or fearful. I ask it because I really want to know the answer. I think it may be years before I truly understand all of the things that have come to me, but I will keep my heart and my eyes open to the possibilities. That's all anyone can really hope to learn in this life—about their true purpose and what it means for them to be here.

At the moment, I just feel lucky to be alive. And lucky is something I haven't felt in a very long time.

Thirteen

Saturday, June 7

6:02 A.M.—I have been awake for an hour now, so I thought I would write as I welcome the day. Since I last wrote, I am further and further away from the completion of my last treatment. With that, there has been endless joy and thanks, as well as anxiety that still hovers near me. Other survivors tell me it's normal.

The lingering side effects from the treatments combined have been minimal, although my heart has raced at times. I am improving each day. This morning when I heard the paperboy, I was unable to go back to sleep. To me it's just a sign that my body has healed enough to greet the day at an earlier hour, no longer needing to sleep so many hours. Even last week, I would be so sound asleep that I wouldn't even hear the mailman long after the paperboy had delivered our newspaper.

Now that I have finished treatment, I still say I would have passed on the entire experience if given the choice, but I try not to dwell on it. As long as I stay well and am able to have children one day, nothing bad has really come from this. There has been suffering, but there has been strength in the weaknesses I've experienced. It has been a difficult journey that I am certain I will have to face all of my life in some capacity, although I pray that the further I travel in my journey, the less I will fear the return of the dysfunction of my body. I build my strength by educating myself with books, people and God.

I don't think about dying anymore. I am not bold enough to say that I am not afraid to die in general. I can say that it is the fear of what can happen while I am living that I must learn to cope with until the process of life and healing teaches me not to fear cancer anymore. I never want to go through the pain I was handed on December 26 and just about everyday since then. Much good has come from something bad, but I hope and expect to learn many lessons from it without having to be shaken again.

The party is today and as I think about the people who are on their way to see me and enjoy the wonderful event that is planned, I am grateful. I wouldn't say that I have lost any friends through this experience, but I have learned who my friends are and watched to see what the weaknesses of others could teach me. I used to spend much of my energy trying to maintain relationships with others who did not make the same efforts, but I no longer do that. The people who have mustered around me through this are the people I will take care of for the rest of my life. Not everyone was able to fully participate in this with my family, but I understand that not everyone can always be awakened at the same time.

When I was nineteen years old and first started college, I baby-sat for a woman named Sue who was undergoing treatment for breast cancer. At the time, I gave her a small card that read: "If you have faith as small as a mustard seed, nothing will be impossible for you." (Matt. 17:20). Soon after I called to tell her that I was diagnosed with Hodgkin's, I received the same card from her. She'd saved it all those years and wanted me to have it. It was one of the most heart-warming gestures I've ever known. My friend Kellee made the cake for my party and wrote the same verse across its top. It's become my motto.

I have felt the presence of Alton in the past few days, even though he has been gone for nearly two years now. I feel like he has known my fate all along and now he sees that I am well again. I like to think that he has watched Wesley become a man through this, and I hope Alton knows how far his son has come. I watch the videos of when Alton was alive, and I see his spirit there. I know how much he loved all of us and I realize what a difference he continues to make in my life. I continue to benefit from the time he spent here, mostly because I get to spend each day of my life with someone he helped create—his son, my husband.

My husband—the hero that I know has rescued me one hundred times or more since the moment we sat in Dr. McCabe's hallway and discovered I had cancer. It was then that we were handed an anchor and an oar and told to sink or swim, grow or wilt, learn or be ignorant, love or be lost. We swam, we grew, we learned and we were found. We literally walked through the valley of the shadow of death and survived, although fearful. We are better for what we have endured. We have strength and we have courage—two qualities that I am sure will continue to grow as we do. We get to be better than we ever thought, as a couple that God brought together and as the individuals God created years ago.

I think about my brother and know that he is a person who strives toward good in his life. I am sure that on many occasions he must have wondered what my illness is meant to teach him. One of the greatest gifts I have been given is my ability to appreciate him. For years I have watched Vance grow into the person he is now, so awake and open in his life. Too many times people live their lives without paying attention. They eat, they drink, they breathe, but they don't really experience any of the gifts that have been laid out for them.

During our many conversations while I was sick, I listened closely to him. I interrupted him at times, but I listened. It was encouraging for me when Vance would call each day to tell me about someone new he had met who knew someone else who had survived Hodgkin's. He and Heather gave me the greatest hope when they sent her Aunt Gina to me.

It's difficult to explain what my coming to know Vance has meant to my life. I cringe at the thought that we might have actually gone through our entire lives without allowing ourselves to experience the love we now hold for each other. He spoke with me, not to me. And many times after reading the book he sent me about creative visualization, I saw him as a silent guide who led me to a window, pulled back the blinds and waited quietly for my eyes to open to a world he had already discovered.

I think that in life there are hopes we have for ourselves, things we desire and things we know we are capable of achieving. And I also think there are things in life that we cannot be sure we will ever attain, but we know we will be better people just by striving for them. I don't think I am supposed to be able to instantly come away from this with great knowledge or wisdom without the work that is ahead of me. That's the beauty of it—we don't have to learn everything at once, we just have to be open to the possibilities of its healing and the people we can become if we are willing to pay closer attention.

I think my brother is one of those people who strive to emulate good in their lives. Truly, all of my family is, and I am thankful for what they have added to my life, to my recovery, and to my beliefs. And as the early morning quiet has passed and we begin to prepare for the party and day of celebration we have all been waiting for, I feel nothing but love for the people who make up my dear family. And all I can hope is that each of them knows that I would have done the same for them—and hopefully just as well.

Sunday, June 8

It was difficult for me to sleep. All I could think about is what a wonderful day it was and how very special I felt to have 108 of the 112 people we invited actually come to the party. It was, by far, one of the best days for my family.

Family and friends traveled from all over the state and other parts of the country to attend. Many of them brought Christmas tree ornaments to hang on the tree my parents bought for the party. My mom thought that since I probably wouldn't read through the cards that people brought very often, I could have the ornaments to hang from my tree each Christmas to remind me of the people who joined us in our celebration. And before Wesley and I leave to go back to Texas, my family will plant the tree in the backyard. It can be a symbol of the life that was saved while we were all home again as a family.

Tracy came from Los Angeles and brought a guest book for people to write in for me. My friend Caroline, who I have known since living next door to her grandma in the house two doors down from ours, brought me purple heart earrings. She said they were a symbol of my bravery.

My dad's best friend since high school, Gary, pulled me aside to say how proud he was of me. He said that my dad went to see him right after I was diagnosed with cancer and asked him to pray for me. I would not consider Gary a religious man, but he knows God and is a man of deep beliefs and convictions. He said that when my dad went to see him he looked more scared and shaken than he had ever seen him. Gary tried to tell my dad not to worry. Gary said: "It was like something inside of me already knew that you were going to be okay. I just knew it. I didn't start to pray for you right away. I waited a few days. Then I got down on my knees near my bed and didn't stand to my feet for five hours. For five hours I prayed for your healing and felt sure that your health would be restored."

There were a number of people whose lives had already encountered cancer before I was diagnosed. Wanda was there and is a four-year survivor of breast cancer. My Uncle Harlow, my grandpa's brother, survived colon cancer, and his other brother, Glenn, survived prostate cancer. My Aunt Pat also came and is a fifteen-year survivor of breast cancer. My dad's friend Randy lost his wife to cancer just last year. He shook Wesley's hand when he thanked us for inviting him. Our friends John and Kirsten were there, and her sister survived Hodgkin's disease several years ago. My friend Darcy drove all the way from Washington for the party. Her dad is a two-time survivor of non-Hodgkin's lymphoma and told me what to expect from my Neupogen shots. There were so many special people there that I could not possibly list them all. But these were the survivors who had more than just my survival to celebrate.

Wesley knew that I had planned to say a few words of thanks to everyone during the party, so he asked me if I wanted to speak to everyone before we all sat down for dinner. I said yes, and before I knew it, all of our guests were gathered around me. And as I looked around at everyone, it occurred to me that I had known most of the people there for more than fifteen years and some for much longer. What a life of stability and love my parents provided for us.

Rod and Cindy, my parents' good friends since I was three years old, came with their family. Rod asked if he could give a prayer before I began. I was honored. He spoke of how long he'd known our family and that he considered Vance and I to be like his own children. He gave thanks for my healing and for the love we could all learn from my family's experience. As he spoke, I thought back to when he came to see me within days after he heard I had cancer. We sat outside and had a private conversation that gave me much strength in the months that lay ahead.

Vance also asked to speak to everyone, but I had to speak after Rod because I was so nervous and thought if I didn't say what I wanted to right then, I might not be able to later. When Vance spoke after me, he talked about how it's not important what kind of car we drive or the house we live in. He said it's lessons like these that define who we are as people. He said that we should appreciate this day, because it turned out the way it did. He said that it could have been a different day, a different reason to gather. I knew what he meant, and it made me feel even better that we had gathered our loved ones. So many times people only gather to celebrate weddings or mourn at funerals. The tears our guests were crying turned to laughter when Vance said, "It's good to learn from these things, I just hope it doesn't have to be this hard again, because I can't handle it."

Mom, Dad, Vance, Heather and Wesley all huddled closely to me. With Wesley holding me tightly while standing at my side and the rest of my family standing close to me, I began to share my feelings of love and restoration with everyone there. I had not written down what I wanted to say, but I had rehearsed the words over and over again in my mind for months. I took a deep breath and began:

I want to thank all of you for coming and tell you that you were invited here today because you contributed in some small or large way to my recovery and my family's sanity over the past six months. It has been a difficult time, but each one of you somehow managed to make it easier.

For several months, I have thought of this day and what I wanted to say to everyone once we gathered here together. It may be difficult, but I want to try and convey my thoughts to you while I have the opportunity.

When we were told I had cancer, it was the most shocking news we had ever received. It took a long time for us to believe it wasn't just a bad dream, because it did not seem real. My dad eventually began calling all of our friends and family, and that started a circle of support that we called upon many times over the months. I'm thankful that we included you in what would have been an even more arduous battle if it had not been for your kindness and prayers.

There are several people I would like to thank. I want to thank Vance for all of his love and support in the past months. Most of you have known us our whole lives and have seen the change in our relationship over the years and especially over the past several months. Vance, your support guided me in times of troubling thoughts, and I thank you for that.

I want to thank my mom for all that she did for me. I was so sick and you fed me bananas when I was too weak to get out of bed, you took my temperature when I was too frightened to, and you rubbed my arm when the medicine hurt. I can't imagine what these months of taking care of your sick child have been like for you, and for this reason alone, I am glad it is over.

I want to thank my dad for changing weekends and coming home when I was sick so he could see what the treatments were like for all of us. I am thankful for the positive presence you were during this, and I want you to know that even though you couldn't always be here,

I knew how important it was for you to be gone working. It enabled us to have more freedom in our time here, and your support of this family helped sustain our stay and allowed me to be home when I needed to be most. I hope that both you and mom will be able to sleep well now and greet each day knowing that you will also have grandpa's good fortune of your children outliving you.

And Wesley—I don't know how to begin to thank you. Wesley and I have talked about this day and wondered which day was most important, our wedding day or this celebration. To us, this day symbolizes our reward for the vows we remained committed to during what was the most difficult time of our marriage. When two people get married, they stand before God and witnesses and pledge their love to one another and make vows that are to be upheld for the rest of their lives. I think when people take those vows, they truly believe in them but are later tested by what they are willing to maintain in their relationship. Wesley and I understood our vows and had already faced challenges with some of them. We understood the richer or for poorer part, because we were students and knew what it was like to struggle. For better or for worse had come to us in our marriage, too. We lost his father. That was the worst. Then there was also better along the way. But the vow about in sickness and in health . . . it's one that many young people never consider and do not have to face for many years.

We were talking with one of my friends recently who was ending a long-term relationship with a man she couldn't imagine spending the rest of her life with. He was a prominent attorney, and they had a lavish lifestyle together, but she said that when they were just at home watching television together, it seemed they had nothing to say to each other. Wesley told her, "Well, you're right to end the relationship if it can't go beyond the excitement of vacations and elaborate meals together, because you never know when you are going to find yourself at home watching television." We laughed at the time, but the more that I thought about it, the more it made perfect sense to me. And that's when it occurred to me how many young people choose their mates. They choose the person they are going to spend the rest of their life with based on where he went to college, if he went to college, or what kind of job he has. These things are important in understanding a person's ambition and level of aptitude, but they tell us nothing about how he will react in a crisis. Wesley has been the most guiding force since this began. I couldn't imagine my life any other way, and I want you to know, Wesley, that I will always do my best to show you how much your love means to me. You saved my life again and again and you are the true definition of a husband.

I also want to thank Bev, Darla and Jeri. I not only want to thank you for going to my treatments and being available to me whenever I needed you, but I also want to thank you for taking your children to chemotherapy. You trusted me to show them a part of the world that wasn't safe or predictable and enabled them to grow as people because of it.

And I want to thank both of my grandmas for caring so much about me. My Grandma Smith called me every day to see how I was feeling, and my Grandma Shaw sent flowers when she knew the treatments were taking their toll on me.

I have to find a way to live the rest of my life without being afraid. I woke up every day and did my best to get well. All of my life I had heard about people who had cancer and what fighters they were. When I got cancer, I started to wonder what this fight was all about. I wondered if it would be something that would come to me like an epiphany, but it didn't. I eventually learned that my fight would be different every day and that some days the fight would be more tiresome and difficult than others. But I made sure that I fought every day, because I wanted to live. I wanted my parents to know that I wanted to survive and make them grandparents. I wanted Wesley to know that I wanted to spend years and years with him, and I wanted to have his children and grow old with him. I needed their help. I needed them to do their part and meet me halfway, so I could do whatever it took. Then win or lose, live or die, they would know I did everything I could to survive. And that's what we did. Every single day.

This has been the hardest thing I have ever had to do. I want this day to be a day of rest and celebration for what we all endured because of cancer. On this day, I close the door and walk through another that leads me to the rest of my life.

While I was speaking, I could hear people crying as they listened. As my family stood huddled together, it seemed, as it should be. When I finished, everyone began to cheer and clap. One guest after the other came to hug us and thank us for inviting them. Many said it was the best party they had ever been to and it was an honor and a privilege to be a part of our celebration and of our lives. When Bev walked over to us, she had a cage with two doves in it. She said she wanted me to set them free as a symbol of letting go of the past six months. And so we did. And as they flew into the sky, I thought about how much I was loved and how good it felt to be alive.

Friday, June 28

Today is the day that I have been both looking forward to and dreading. Today we go back to Texas. The car is already packed and we have said most of our good-byes.

I went to see both Dr. Verma and Dr. McCabe. Dr. Verma had ordered blood work and a chest X-ray and told me during our visit that the tests proved I was in remission. I wrote each of them letters of thanks. I thanked Dr. McCabe for looking after me and for sending me to Dr. Verma.

In my letter to Dr. Verma, I thanked him for being instrumental in saving my life and for taking every precaution to not over-toxify my young body. I gave him a picture frame that I made for him and asked that he put it in his office to make it more inviting to the new patients that would come through his door. Kim said that Dr. Verma was very touched by what I'd written in the card. He told her, "This is very emotional for me." I felt happy to have made a doctor emotional about his patient.

Jeri and my grandmas were here earlier to say good-bye. Bev is still here. She will be here until we pull out of the driveway and are out of sight. That's Bev, there for me until the very end. Others have also come to say good-bye. My parents have written in my got-well party guest book. I will always treasure their words on this day that I must leave here for what I know is the final time. I know I will never live in this house again. Honestly, I don't think I'd want to. It is time for me to move forward and embrace Texas and all that it holds there for us. In the past, I have always felt lonely for this part of my life, but I think now I will simply consider my home to be wherever Wesley and I are together.

I spent a week with my brother and Heather after the party and aside from Vance getting frustrated with me for not attempting to climb a hill that was ten blocks high, we had a wonderful visit. When he said that I should at least try, I started to cry. I told him, "I know that from the outside I look like I am in perfect health. My hair is growing back, my eyes no longer have dark circles and I feel much better. But you weren't there, and you just don't know how hard it is to get it all back. You didn't see it." He felt badly and went to get the car. We walked and walked, but up ten blocks I could not go.

Vance and Heather came back last weekend to say good-bye. It was difficult for us to part, but the tears I cried felt like years of relief for what we had come away with. In a card he gave to me he wrote: "I love you, Lisa. And now that we know more about what that really means, that's all I will say."

My parents, Wesley and I have spent much of the day talking about the past months. My dad has been wearing his sunglasses, even while inside the house. It's difficult for him to show his tears, but he knows he is not hiding what he feels in his heart. I worry about my parents after I leave, because I know they will be saddened. But I also know what my mom has said again and again: "When you and Vance are happy, we are happy."

So many things change inside of me each day while I wait for peace to come in the times that I pray for it. I make my search every day from the place I live, the heart that heals, and the mind that wants to let go of everything that brings it back. I know that it will eventually get easier and the times in between the pain will be farther apart. The faith I have always known will have lifted me out of this darkness that I now realize I have not yet completely moved away from. Light surrounds me and leads my way, but that pure pleasure of believing it every minute of every day still awaits me.

I continue to feel rescued. Wesley continues to rescue me. And when the panic comes over my face and stirs up the bad things inside of my heart, he says to stop, to be grateful, and to trust in everyone and everything that healed me—

including myself. And then I return. I return from that place where everything is confused and wrong in the world since hearing the word cancer, and I am rescued in the hope that what we did worked. And I realize that people spent years of their lives learning about cancer and its treatments so I could have a chance to survive.

In my strength I can now think of my grandpa and not shed tears of longing. I may hurt less than I did when he first died, but that is only because I have a better understanding of his departure and how times heals the things that would otherwise destroy us. My dad's oldest sister, my Aunt Jo, told me as she was leaving the party that she thought of Grandpa a lot while I was sick and that I was just like him. If I have managed to gain even a seed of his wisdom in my journey, then I have learned beyond my years. I know he would be proud of me today.

There was so much of him in my spirit that kept me fighting. I used to watch him silently sit when he had cancer. I wondered if he was in pain, because he would never show it. He just stood like the pillar of our family and protected us from what was coming. I have no doubt that any pain he experienced while sick with cancer would not have amounted to the pain he would have known watching me have it. I am thankful his life was spared suffering through it. He got to leave this earth never watching any of his offspring suffer illness or pain.

I think of him differently now than I did before I got sick. I think about what caused him to die and know that I also walked the path of cancer, only my walk will be longer. I feel like I have a closeness with him that no one else in our family can comprehend. It's like I am standing on the inside with him while those we love are standing outside of us.

I remember listening to him on the telephone when he was diagnosed with cancer. He was making calls to find out how much money my grandma would continue to receive after he died. I was amazed by his strength and being able to courageously say that he had a terminal illness and wanted to make sure his wife would be taken care of after he died. He and my grandma were married for fifty-two years, had five children, eleven grandchildren, and a growing family of great-grandchildren. Cancer didn't take that man's life, because he had already taken everything he possibly could from life.

I loved my grandpa, and I still do today. I don't believe that just because a person dies our love for him has to stop growing. If anything, my love has continued to grow for him because I have a better understanding of his purpose and of his significance in my life. I know Wesley will love his father even more when he has a son of his own because of all that he will discover about himself as a father.

I never told Wesley or my parents, but when I was first diagnosed my determination to survive was guided by two very specific reasons. I refused to let my parents bury me, and I refused to make Wesley a widower at twenty-seven years old.

I don't think any parent is equipped to cope with the loss of a child. I have seen the suffering that always follows when the natural order is destroyed. All I could imagine was my mom living her life in a crumbled state and my father spending the rest of his life trying to suppress his pain so that he could help fill the void in my mother's heart. I could not even see Wesley surviving it. I do not say that because I would be beyond replacing in his life, because many people who lose their spouses eventually find a way to go on with their lives and choose a new person to share it with. I say it because Wesley had already suffered enough in his life, and if I died, especially so soon after his father, he would question what in his life was worth living for. I didn't want his life to be tainted by my death and all that would come with it.

I never told any of them these thoughts, because I knew they would dismiss them mainly out of fear and also to try and make me feel better. I kept these thoughts to myself, and when things seemed unbearable, I thought about what I had to do to spare them the suffering of my untimely death. As morbid as it may seem, it was enough to help me fight harder when I felt like it was a losing battle. And now I see that it gave me strength and it empowered me. However they may have tried to stop me from thinking that way, it worked and I fought hard because of it.

Somewhere in between all that happened to me before this and all that has happened to me since then, I feel like there is something waiting—something I am to accomplish, to help others, to help myself, and to put the pieces back together.

I thought I was as strong as I could possibly be when I stood in front of our family and friends at my party and thanked them for what they contributed to my recovery, but I continue to get stronger in my walk through this spooky layer of fear. I do what I am told, remaining compliant, ever hoping that doing what is best will help sustain my life. It's all become about sustaining my life, about having the chance to give life, and about realizing what my life is to mean—what I am to accomplish.

In the words of my Aunt Jeri from a page in my guest book: "I believe you were selected to learn and to teach us all to trust in not only ourselves, but also in God. . . . Life is a classroom with many lessons to learn. It's time you graduated from this one and on to another. I know the next one will be more fun."

Fourteen

Thoughts from My Father

I asked my dad to give me some of the journal entries he had written after I recovered. When I read his pages, I cried. This is what he wrote:

I thought Lisa's itching was something minor and a bit overstated. I figured her other symptoms were probably just flu-like, winter's malady of ills, aches and pains. When she asked me to call Dr. McCabe to make an appointment the day after Christmas, she had me feel a lump in her neck. Swollen glands, we assessed. Something in my heart raced, but it was not despair and not much more than concern. I figured she would see the doctor and would be okay.

When I called to make the appointment on a Tuesday morning, God must have had someone cancel his or her appointment, because Lisa could see Dr. McCabe that day. He is a busy man, with a thriving practice. He loves my children. He brought them into the world. I have no doubt he became a doctor just for times like these and people like us. I'm sure at times we all run together just like another day at the office, but not on this day. On this day, he was the first to begin putting the pieces of this puzzle together. Concern became action, course and direction. Damn, we were babes in the woods. We knew nothing of this type of threat.

We are a family of four: father, mother, son and daughter. And in the years we have been together, each of us has grown into individuals that make me proud as the father of this family. We are proud of our children, who do, in fact, exceed our capabilities. Isn't that the goal of parenting? Faster, stronger, smarter, and, if this world is to flourish, wiser.

Lisa called from her appointment terribly upset. She needed Wesley there with her and asked me to bring him. After I hung up the phone, her mother and I looked at each other, but quickly put aside what could be the worst-case scenario. Nothing terrible could happen.

I think my mind was coping well, and I was able to keep my senses. The threats of my deepest despair tried to invade my thoughts. But I told myself, "No, not now. You must tell yourself this will turn out to be the best case. Surely that is what we will deal with."

By the time Lisa and Wesley got home from the doctor, I saw in her something more devastating than I can explain. She managed to speak the words, "He thinks it's cancer." The look in her mother's eyes was instantaneous and absolute devastation. Carmen would have crumbled had we not held each other. We literally held each other up. Our knees were weak; our hearts were in agony.

I can remember looking and not seeing. Not because of the torrent of tears, but because the fear and despair left me void of continuous thought. It was trying to consume us. "No, not now," I told myself again.

After the lymph node biopsy two days later, we went as a family to Dr. McCabe's office to face whatever this was. Wesley and Lisa sat huddled in fear. We all held each other, trying to convince ourselves it was just a bad dream. Dr. McCabe was soon standing with us, verifying what Lisa had tried to tell us after seeing him the first day. The tests were in; it was cancer. Lisa had Hodgkin's disease.

My daughter had cancer. This is the young woman who set out to take this life of hers and share it with a person who, I guess, she had loved since she was eight years old. Maybe I was a little jealous that he could mean that much to her. She turned everything upside down and went and got him. It was torpedoes full-speed ahead for her when she found Wesley. He didn't have a chance, because Lisa was young, beautiful and she loved him. She was the woman he'd always wanted and just didn't know it yet. Maybe God knew that Wesley was the one to be there when this came to her life.

When they first got together I had my doubts, but everybody is wrong at times. He stood by, held up, loved, and even carried my daughter when only the man she shared her life with could. He could have been less wonderful. He could have been just ordinary. He even could have given up and left, but he didn't. He did every man proud, and I love him for that. He is, after all, his father's son. What's not to love?

I have thought of Alton during this and knew how proud he must be of the man his son has become. Alton lived long enough to see Wesley and Lisa together and I thank God for that, because he loved my daughter like his own.

As I listened to Dr. McCabe confirm that Lisa had Hodgkin's and not non-Hodgkin's lymphoma, I found its meaning in his eyes. This was here, it was absolute, and nothing could make it not happen. He had told us to pray for Hodgkin's in the two days before the biopsy, so that is what I accepted first. No mistakes were made. We had to fight this, and non-Hodgkin's scared me to mush, because I saw whatever it was all over her X-ray. But right then, I accepted either.

The drive home from the doctor's office was surreal. We grouped ourselves together enough to present the most appropriate parents for Lisa's sake. Time sort of passed slowly that evening. My emotions took me two steps forward and then two steps backward. The reality shook us all and rattled our spirits.

We've all had trying times in our lives, but this was a glimpse at personal holocaust. This was my daughter. I had thoughts of fear—fear of being destroyed. My father never suffered through this. What a gift. Whenever the kids were late getting home, I never thought the worst. I'd tell their mother they were out being kids and they'd get home safely. I was always right. But what was this? This was something I couldn't control. This was like the phone call every parent dreads getting.

That night, her mother and I lay in bed and cried as we held onto each other. I could feel Carmen trembling. Sleep eventually came to us. Looking back it must've seemed like a long, solid sleep. When I woke up it was 11:45 P.M. I really just sat straight up in bed. Whether I woke up on my own, or my wife woke me, I do not remember. I believe that God woke me to tell me that Lisa was going to be okay. I knew this to be the truth. It wasn't like I had to convince anyone else or myself of it. As surely as it had happened, I knew it was going to be okay. My daughter was not only going to survive, but she was going to flourish. My father's gift was mine; my daughter was going to outlive me and have a long and wonderful life. The order was back. The certainty had returned.

Carmen immediately began to educate herself about Lisa's cancer. She wanted to be prepared for what lay ahead. Carmen has this amazing ability to put herself aside and focus on others. I truly admired her deeds in the times ahead. Her selflessness was abundant. I'd come home and push my optimism on her, Wesley and Lisa, then I'd go back to work and leave them with the uncertainty of the next day and the days after. But Carmen stayed and lived only to take care of our daughter.

In the days after Lisa was diagnosed, I was driving down the freeway. My thoughts were racing. I thought of everything pertinent and everything not. And suddenly I lost my resolve. Fear, despair and devastation took over again. I could not fathom my existence without Lisa. My daughter had cancer. She could die. Her mother would never be the same. How would I ever enjoy life's little treasures? Everyday, Lisa would be gone. I've lost my father, but that's okay, because he didn't lose me. I've lost two of my best friends and how I miss them, but I could not even accept the possibility of losing my daughter.

As I drove along the freeway in the pouring rain, I had to pull over to the side of the road. I had to literally slap myself. "No, not now. Not these thoughts." Damn, I lose again. I had never known such total lack of control. I was sobbing.

Somehow, after what seemed an eternity of despair, I was blessed to feel God help me pull myself together.

This happened to me more than once over the course of our battle against cancer. Yes, I had some doubts, but the overwhelming thoughts, the ones I could feel when I took deep breaths to cleanse my mind and my spirit told me that everything was going to be okay.

I remember it as if we were all on these separate islands all by ourselves, dealing with this in our own way. But at the same time, we were holding on to the same island of hope. After Lisa saw the filthy and vile cancer they took from her body, I could see the pain in my baby girl's eyes. She was being so brave.

I believe Lisa thought my reaction to her diagnosis was strange. Maybe it was just my perception, but I believe Dr. McCabe beamed with relief when the lump proved to be Hodgkin's disease. Lisa gasped in despair. Wesley sank. Her mother sat in disbelief. I rejoiced; God and I had already worked it out. "No, not despair. This was the best-case scenario." This was God's first gift toward the return of my daughter's life. It was totally curable. And at that moment, the forces of faith and family began to work.

The conversation I'd had with God was racing through my mind while I listened to the doctor address our questions and concerns. Still, I had thoughts of victory instilled in my mind. The physical battle, the drain of spirit, the rise of spirit and the tenacity of Lisa's will and all that loved her were going to triumph. We had Hodgkin's. It was going to lose. Dr. McCabe had come to us with the truth and the conviction we needed in order to win. So then we began to rally. Cancer could not have Lisa. Hide and watch, my daughter will win.

We started to gather our army of friends and family. I got on the phone and called each person Lisa asked me to. One after the next spoke in shock as they offered their support and prayers. We even had angels in those who had already passed. We would not be let down.

I remember calling my mother—she lost most of her voice as a child because of medication for narcolepsy and I hear so-so at best, but her voice was clear and disbelieving. She just didn't want to believe it. Not her granddaughter. I wondered how long after we hung up it took to really sink in. My mom must have cried alone in her bed that night—or my dad's spirit lifted her a bit, didn't it?

It's been a long time since the cancer came into and left our lives. Yesterday, my little girl went to the cancer center for a check-up. I know it is bittersweet to her, more bitter than sweet. The check-ups confirm her good health, but they also bring back the reality of the past in the black hole of cancer. She had it, and I'm sure sporadically the memories and fears slip into her conscious thoughts.

Her mother and Wesley were there for chemo and the daily stress of it all, so were some really special people that Lisa chose to include. And yes, I drove or flew home to be there for her chemo weekends. But Lisa was the only one with cancer in her body. She sometimes gets irritated with me because I only think positively in certain situations, but she only has to look in the mirror to see the most determined positive thinker she will know in her life.

I know I rarely let doubt creep in, but I wasn't sick and tired from being physically poisoned. Did she lay in her bed and feel the battle her mind and spirit were waging against this disease? How did she put aside twitches and pains or maybe something she could feel last week but was later gone? Did she know she was winning? Oh yes, she did. But that couldn't remove the doubts and fears.

Sometimes I saw her so close to being overwhelmed, so I would just hug or talk to her and try to bring her thoughts away from that place. But how many times weren't we there? Lisa had so many countless battles to wage and win just to keep her spirit and confidence to defeat her perverse enemy. She had to stay strong and get stronger as needed—like during the days leading up to her next chemo treatment—she couldn't face dread constantly. How wonderful it is that God lets strong people put aside that dread for periods of time. Her reserve turned into fortitude, fortitude to further strength, and strength into life. My little girl fought a monster and she won. My daughter faced cancer and the realities that came with it and she prevailed.

Lisa asked me to shave her head while she was sick. Looking back, although it made her look different and everyone could see that she was sick, after she got used to it I think it was a confidence-builder. She almost acted like the little girl in the big sunglasses when she was a kid. She didn't care if anyone stared. She just stared back. It was almost like her badge of courage for all to see.

Her life has gone on now. Everyone survived, and I thank God for that every day. I don't go to church, but I have always believed in good and believe a man who had God in his life with or without the structure of a church or of religion can have the gift of eternity. My daughter proves that.

Fifteen

Three Years Later

May, 1999

As much as I wanted to believe that I would be able to close the door to cancer and walk through the rest of my life unscathed by what it had done to me, both physically and emotionally, it would prove to be the most difficult task.

In the early weeks after returning to Texas, I think I adapted well to the realities of everyday life. In fact, I welcomed the routines that we fell back into when we went back to our normal lives. I became frustrated when certain things became too routine, like when Wesley and I argued about the dishes or other ridiculous things. I didn't understand or welcome it after having just saved my life, but I also understood that some of the tedious things in life would return, as would the frustration of getting them done.

Other things I didn't expect occurred. Shortly after radiation ended, I developed a dry cough. I was nervous about going to a doctor about it, but I forced myself. For the first time since having cancer, I had to fill out a routine questionnaire in the doctor's office. It saddened me when I had to check the box marked "cancer." It was one month before my twenty-fifth birthday, and as much as I welcomed the coming year, I was reminded of what a fragile young life was mine. Although, this time, I did simply get medicine and go home. The cough persisted for several weeks, but it diminished with time, as did my compulsion to check for lumps.

It wasn't until my first check-up at the end of September 1996 that I really had a breakdown. I remember having trouble breathing during my only panic attack. Wesley and I were standing in the kitchen, and he had to grab me by my shoulders and shout at me to calm down. I was terrified of returning to be checked for cancer, and it wasn't making it any easier to be going to a new doctor and hospital to have the tests done.

When Wesley and I arrived at the hospital, I was assigned a patient advocate, who helped in making me feel like more than just a number, but it was nothing like where I had been treated. It may have had the best of some things, but I thanked God once again for placing me in Dr. McCabe's hands when I found the lump in my neck. Being treated in California was best for me. I knew I had to move on and do my follow-up elsewhere, but it was difficult to start anew.

Because I was a new patient, my oncologist, Dr. Younes, insisted that I repeat numerous tests so they could establish their own baseline, including a bone marrow biopsy. When I read the order on the paper, I immediately began to cry. I told Wesley I was getting on a plane and going back to Dr. Verma. Over the next several days before the tests were to begin, Sue, my patient advocate, called me at home and tried to convince me to repeat the tests. Without all of them, Dr. Younes would not be able to give me the "remission" word, and as much as

I hated to admit it, I would need it for my medical status.

Sue said that they could prescribe a sedative for me to take before the bone marrow biopsy to help me relax, and so after numerous conversations with her, Wesley, God and myself, I agreed to take the sedative and have the biopsy. After all of the times I refused sedatives during treatment, I decided it was time to be physically numbed in order to move forward. I'd suffered enough pain in the months before; I was done being the pillar of strength. I didn't feel weak, I just felt resolve.

The sedative didn't help the pain entirely, but it helped me relax before and after. It was just as painful as the first time. Only this time, someone did it whose job it was to do the biopsy every day. It was done more quickly but not less painfully.

When the results to all of the tests came back negative, particularly the bone marrow biopsy, I wanted to say, "I told you so," but I didn't. I just agreed to be back in three months for more tests.

I have continued to go for check-ups as they are scheduled. I went every three months the first year, every four months the second, and every six months the third. At no time since the clear gallium scan that enabled me to stop chemotherapy has there ever been a question about my remission status. I have been cancer-free for more than three years.

There have been times over the past three years that I have been faced with many aspects of healing that I had not expected. For the most part, Wesley moved on from cancer the day we drove away from my parents' house and headed for Texas. He listened and supported me through the difficulty I had in finding my way through the thick fear that hovered over me for months, even years to come long after he moved on.

The first October following treatment was a month spent in absolute fear, because I had to hear the word *cancer* over and over again. Breast Cancer Awareness month brings about awareness for all of the right reasons, but for those of us who know what cancer means and what it can do, it's hard to get away from. The Octobers since the first have gotten increasingly easier. I can watch and listen and not feel the doom of another cancer that could happen to me. I have learned to live my life in a way that empowers me against these things and lends to my mental, physical and spiritual stability.

Perhaps the survivorship I have experienced with other survivors has been among the most rewarding. I've had the opportunity to meet numerous people who also survived and it's a commonality that I hold dear. For many check-ups, I have been the youngest patient in the room, but amongst the other survivors, I was just that—a survivor.

I remember when I was going through treatment and former patients would tell me about their experiences with cancer, they would sometimes have to count the years back out loud to remember exactly when it had occurred. I thought that was amazing and the first time it happened to me, I wanted to cry. I felt freedom from it in a way I hadn't expected.

For many months after being diagnosed, I wondered what my life would have been like if the cancer had never come. When I sat in a waiting room for my check-ups, I would wonder what I might have been doing on that day if I'd never had cancer. Nothing in my life changed that train of thought, until July 13, 1998. On that day, everything changed.

It had been more than two years since I had been told that my cancer was in remission. During that time, the doctors told Wesley and I to wait at least one year before trying to have a baby, and they said that two years would be even better, because the threat of recurrence would be drastically reduced. We were told that it might be difficult to get pregnant, maybe even impossible. Because I never went back on birth control pills and we had only been practicing natural methods of birth control, we assumed they were right and thought our chances of conceiving a child were hindered by the treatments I'd endured. When asked if we wanted to have tests done to check for estrogen levels and other fertility indicators, we refused, once again leaving it up to God.

On several occasions in the second year of my remission, I tried convincing Wesley that we should start trying to have a baby in case it took us years to actually get pregnant. I even suggested that we get on an adoption waiting list early on, in case our attempts were not successful. He refused both suggestions and remained ever faithful to his role, as the man who believed everything would work out for the best.

We waited until June of 1998 to try and get pregnant. I knew that if we tried in the first year of my recovery, I would worry too much about cancer and not be able to focus on the joy of my pregnancy. The doctors suggested I wait for physical reasons, but what that did was give me one more year to trust in my body and its capabilities. Over the two years of check-ups, I had taken several pregnancy tests to make sure I was not pregnant before having CAT scans, and I always made the technician shield my lower body when having a chest X-ray. I remained ever careful to help ensure our chances.

It was a Monday afternoon on July 13, and I had expected my period to start on the previous Friday morning. I was very regular, so being three days late was unusual, but I didn't really think I could be pregnant because we had only been trying to conceive for one month. But a little voice inside of me kept saying that a miracle was beginning. Wesley and I had done all of the other pregnancy tests together, but this time, I just stopped at the grocery store on my way home and bought a test and a roll of film. Wesley was still at work, and I didn't even tell him that I'd bought it.

When I got home, I started dinner, got myself together and

headed for the bathroom. I had taken enough tests to know that waiting for the stick to give results was maddening, so I did the test, set the timer for three minutes and left the room. It was a long three minutes, but I made myself stay out of the bathroom until the alarm rang.

Finally, the sound of the alarm allowed me to enter the bathroom. I picked up the stick and, at first, saw nothing. For a brief second, I felt a sense of emptiness in the pit of my stomach, but as I began to leave the bathroom, I looked again at the result stick. And there it was. It was faint and hard to see, but the line across the result window could not be mistaken. It was positive; I was pregnant!

I started to walk in circles, not really knowing where I was heading. Then suddenly, as I was walking out our bedroom door, I dropped to my knees and began to sob. As I cried out loud, I began to speak to God. I wanted to give thanks in that moment for what I had been given. I wanted to shout it from the rooftops that I had been given a second miracle. As the emotions stirred inside of me, I thought about how far I'd come. I thought about how blessed I was that the same body that had created something as horrible as cancer had now created something as miraculous as a human life.

Truly, there has never been a more defining moment for me then the day I discovered I was pregnant. Again, something had come to my life and in an instant everything had changed, and I became someone so different than I was before. When I dropped to my knees and cried and thanked God, I knew what was coming . . . redemption. From that moment on, after years of feeling like there was a haunting inside that had to slowly heal, I had no fear. Every hurt and every distrust in my body, everything that was ever bad fell away, and I was left with the perfect thought of our baby. My vision was clear, my purpose was clear, and on that day I became a mother.

As the tears fell, I thought about Wesley and how happy he would be. I thought about my parents and what joy this would bring them. I thought about the others, the people who had stood by us during our battle against cancer and who knew how much we wanted a baby. I thought about Wesley and I and how much we wanted to be parents and what good parents we would be.

As these thoughts ran wildly through my mind, I quickly ran to the kitchen and grabbed the roll of film I had purchased when buying the pregnancy test. I wanted to tell Wesley in a unique way, so I wrapped the result stick in a box and decided to give it to him as soon as he got home. I had the camera ready to capture his reaction.

When he got home, I managed to carry on idle conversation until he got settled in, but within a few minutes of him entering the house, I had given him the box to open. I stood with the camera ready while he opened the box. At first, he thought it strange that I'd wrapped up a new toothbrush for him, but then he took a closer look. And click! There was the perfect photo of a father-to-be standing with his jaw to the floor and a positive pregnancy test in his hand. It was, for us, the most perfect discovery.

We spent the next two nights calling all of our family and friends to share the good news. We were endlessly overwhelmed with delight and amazement. I immediately began a calculated search for the perfect obstetrician and, once again, was blessed with a doctor who wanted nothing but the best of care for me. I had scheduled visits with numerous doctors. She was the first one I met with and I canceled all of my other appointments after leaving her office, because she was exactly what I was looking for. Dr. Julie Bernell was the perfect doctor to care for us and get us safely to the miracle birth of our baby.

In our first meeting, I insisted that Dr. Bernell not treat me any differently because of my medical history. I told her I did not want my pregnancy to be tainted by cancer. She agreed, but being the thorough doctor she was, she went above and beyond to look after me and the baby. As much as I fought her on some things, like the second-level ultrasound that she ordered for no other reason than my medical history, I knew she was just looking out for us.

Wesley and I went through Lamaze because we both wanted me to be able to deliver our baby naturally. I had been through pain before without any reward, so I knew that I could get through it. I knew that I wanted to feel the entire experience and not be numbed to the pain so that I might fully know the joy. For me, there was no other option.

The weeks turned into months, and finally the day arrived. My mom had come from Oregon two weeks before my due date, because most of the babies on my mother's side arrived two weeks early, including my brother and me. We were as prepared as we could be when I went into labor twelve days before our baby was due.

The day our baby was born began as any other day. It was a Monday morning and Wesley was just about to leave for the office when I started having a painful contraction. I had been having pre-labor contractions all weekend, but this one felt different than those. Wesley sat with me through the contraction, and when it was almost over, I told him to take me to the hospital. I knew it was time.

I spent my whole life preparing for this task . . . for the miracle of our baby. People said I was crazy to want to go through childbirth without an epidural to numb the pain, but I knew that I wanted to experience our baby completely. With Wesley's help, we brought our child into this world in the truest way we knew how. And after twelve hours of labor, our baby was born. We had a son. We named him Hunter Alton after Wesley's father and knew that God had given us a second chance when he gave us our son. Immediately after he was born, Wesley held me for several minutes and would not let go of his embrace. We cried tears of joy, tears of relief and tears of redemption, because in the moment Hunter was born, I was healed.

Our mothers were in the delivery room when Hunter was born. They both were very supportive and helpful. All modesty disappeared when it came time to deliver our baby, and having Donna on one side of me and Wesley on the other helped me feel more comfortable. Sharing that experience with Wesley's mom and knowing that Roger was on the other side of the doors waiting, I felt closer to the two of them than ever before. I looked forward to the years our baby would spend with his Nana and Papa. My father was listening on the telephone throughout the entire delivery. I think of all the things I could say about my parents, the most important thing would be that they have been waiting for Hunter their entire existence. He is the jewel in their crown. It scares me to think about what this world might be like for him when he is my age, but I think that the most important thing his dad and I can do for our son is what my parents did for me . . . love him unconditionally. I knew there was nothing my brother or I could do to relinquish that love. It was everlasting.

There were times over the years that it seemed our family was on the brink of destruction, but in the end, the one important vessel remained—my parents' commitment. My grandpa once said that priorities were the secret to his family's longevity—and not just his immediate family, but also the families that would carry on after him. My grandparents laid a foundation for what would follow, and it's partly because of them that my own parents' marriage survived the lean years.

I know that my dad will spend years teaching Hunter things

about the great outdoors, the game of golf and everything else he's come to enjoy in his fifty years. My mom will be the one of the two making sure he is always safe during these ventures. It's always been her job to worry out of love and his to reassure out of faith—faith that nothing truly bad could ever happen to this family. And now, despite the bad that did come, Hunter is the good that made it all worth it.

I've asked them to have Hunter call them Grandpa and Grandma to represent the simplicity of two people who were good parents and will be equally grand in their new role. Hunter is their gift for the years they spent building this family; honoring their commitment and letting the difficult things fall away. My parents get to truly reap the rewards of their dedication over the years. They remained committed to each other, to our family and now to their grandson. It truly is the most enduring evolution. It is a cycle that God has always intended for us to experience while we are here on this great planet. It is, my family—and beyond that, there isn't much more a boy could ask for.

I look back at the years Wesley and I have spent together and so many things have become clear in our pursuit of happiness in our new family. There were times when Wesley may have thought he was undeserving of the loyalty I always gave him, but we all fall short of what we think deserves redemption in life. And the principle behind anything that is to last is the commitment we are willing to give it, the time we are willing to allow it, and the truth we find in it for ourselves. There has never been anything but truth in the way Wesley and I have loved each other. Many question whether or not love at first sight is even possible, but I do not. I think love at first sight is just a love that is deemed possible of wonderful things. What comes from that love is always only determined by what is given to it in the choices later made.

In many ways, Wesley is very complicated; but in others, he

is very simple. Give him still waters and a fishing pole and he's happy for hours. He is centered by the time he spends outdoors and is driven by the times in between. My husband is a stand-up guy and no one knows that better than I do. He took care of me when I needed him most and his loyalty during that time was admired by many. He loves his family and has a vivid understanding of what works in maintaining a family and what falls short of that. There is nothing he could have ever wanted more than to be able to provide the life that he and I have always wanted for ourselves—and now the life that we want for our son.

I am now in a place in my life where I truly have no complaints. And where Wesley and I have ended up is nothing short of a gift from God. The two of us have each experienced trials in our lives that made us question whether or not this type of contentment was even possible, but I think those trials have made this place all the better.

The greatest rewards in life come when we are receiving of them. As I sit here and write these words, I am completely aware of the fact that getting everything I ever wanted in life is not what is most important. What is most important is *realizing* that I got everything I ever wanted in life.

Sometimes when Wesley is sitting across the room from me, I look over at him when he does not notice and just marvel in the joy that I experience being with him now. All I ever wanted was to spend my days with him, making a family and a life that we could be proud of. And now, each day that is what I do. I think it's nothing short of wonderful when he enters a room and to this day, I still feel like a kid at heart when he is near. When he is away, I lack something that is only retrieved when he returns. And that, I have discovered, is love.

It's the simplicities of life that I have come to see so clearly after almost losing my life. It's a gift I never intend to take for granted. I think it allows me to see for myself what will always come first and what will be secondary to that. And this family will always come first.

Over the years, I have come to understand that there are a few constants in my life that have enabled me to trust in many things and venture out into a world that may have otherwise seemed unsafe. I have always had a mom and dad who love each other; a brother who, although very different from me, has the most important thing in common with me—we both come from Mick and Carmen Shaw; and Wesley, who I have known most of my life and loved all of that time. It's because of these things that I am able to be who I am and to share these lessons with our son. It was my parents who gave me this life and it is Wesley who helps sustain it—and now there is Hunter.

It has been more than two months since the day he was born, and this is the first chance I have really had to write these words. It seems fitting that it has taken me this long, because the joy of bringing him into the world with his father is difficult to express with words.

During the simplest times of the day—during his bath or while he sleeps or even when he cries because he is hungry, mad or tired—all I can see in him is the love I have waited for all of my life. I saw his dad for the first time when I was a little girl and have always loved him, but it seems that bringing our child into this world together has given me even more to love. Our son, alone, has enabled me to expand my capacity for love. I see things in his father I didn't know were there. I see him in our son—in his face, in his body and even in his temper. Much of this is genetics, but most of it is just the observation of a mother who waited her whole life for all she has now.

I always wanted to be a mother. I wanted to raise children and try to teach them what I learned and give them the skills to learn even more. They say it should be each parent's goal to enable their children to exceed their own capabilities and to give them what they need in order to accomplish the tasks at hand, to excel in life, and to be good people. If Wesley and I accomplish that as parents, I will be proud for what we brought to Hunter's life. And in the years we spend trying, I look forward to waking up every day and looking into the eyes of the little boy we created and saying, "Teach me something again today. Teach me how to help you grow."

At first I questioned whether or not I should even mention the word *cancer* in my words to Hunter when he grows older, but I just don't see any way around explaining my transition, my metamorphosis. Cancer is, by definition, the worst word there is in my opinion. It's powerful, and it has a way of changing lives in the instant it is discovered. And in that moment, the moment that it crept into our lives, I thought I was lost forever. I thought there would be no redemption. During the battle, I feared the worst and I fought everyday for what I hoped would be a full recovery. Wesley helped me, my parents helped us, and so many others were there to help lead the way. And as we all moved through it, I began to pay attention to the things in my life that were changing. Once I did finally recover, I quickly realized that the fear would remain for a long time to come. Nothing seemed to ease my doubt for long—the fear continued to linger. It lingered until Hunter.

I sometimes think about other people who have cancer and try to send them thoughts of strength, wisdom and guidance. Where there is weakness, strength can be found and can help lift others to a place where peace and trust are waiting.

I pray that those who are battling cancer will hold on to what gives them strength and that they'll discover their lives can be enriched by what they can learn from their own cancer experience. I wish them peace and comfort in the places they go in their lives, in their hearts and in their minds.

Cancer cells are not strong ones that overpower all that is good in one's body. They are weak cells that are unsure of their purpose and multiply. There is so much cancer cannot do. I pray for others to seek those things, find those things and live those things. I pray that others will look for the light at the end of this dark tunnel and, hopefully, light will be found in places that they never thought to look.

I am blessed to know that there is no longer cancer inside of me and there hasn't been for years. And for those who share my good fortune, I embrace each one of them. I hold them close in my heart for the rest of my life. For the journey we have traveled and the battle we have won makes us stronger, more faithful people than we were before. May we continue to pay attention to the things that brought us here—to this place of healing and desired peace. May we always remember what we have gained and let go of what was lost and be better because of it. And may we always lift others who find themselves in the path that we have already walked, for we all will have struggled and we all will have gained enough to give something back.

While I was sick, many people told me that my life would be restored after I recovered from cancer, but I never believed them until I opened myself up to the possibilities. Cancer isn't the worst thing that can happen to a person, but it is the worst thing that ever happened to me. And learning to live beyond the words of being told I had cancer seemed impossible at times, but I did it.

I never knew that I was capable of knowing such complete and utter peace in my life. Its rewards are beyond my own comprehension at times, but I remain ever grateful. It took years of healing and restoration, but now I have managed to turn cancer into something more than a devastating diagnosis and into something that had to happen in order for me to receive the gifts that have belonged to me since then.

Time is, in fact, the great healer I had always heard it to be. And in the time I have spent overcoming the hurt that cancer brought to my life, I have come to believe that I am worthy of the happiness I now know. If all that I was ever given after being freed of cancer was the gift of our son, then surely that would have been enough.

I now know that, although some things in my life have been difficult, all things have led me to Hunter. And honestly, I would live every day of my life exactly the same if it meant creating him all over again. Because more than the reason I survived, he is the reason I was born.

About the Author

Lisa Shaw-Brawley was diagnosed with Hodgkin's disease at the age of twenty-four and learned firsthand about the ordeal of treatment and the common physical and emotional stages of recovery. Her articles related to cancer research and recovery have appeared in Houston's *Sun* and *Observer* newspapers.

Lisa speaks with cancer patients and to related organizations about her own cancer experience and overcoming the risk of infertility.

A senior and a journalism major at Texas A&M University, Lisa is currently on hiatus from school while staying at home to raise her son. She lives with her family in Texas.

To contact Lisa, send an email to *CancerJourneys@aol.com.*

A portion of the author's proceeds will be donated to MD Anderson Cancer Center, benefitting cancer research.

Words and Pictures to Inspire Your Spirit

Second Thoughts

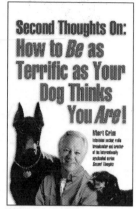

In this touching selection of essays, journalist and speaker Mort Crim shares the lessons he learned from his dogs and the comfort they brought into his life. From welcoming him home from work each day to helping him through the death of his first wife, his animals shared canine love and wisdom in ways that will touch-and sometimes break-your heart.

Code #7842 • Quality Paperback • $12.95

Wyland Ocean Wisdom

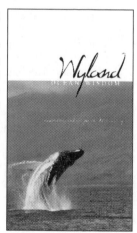

In this beautifully illustrated book, critically acclaimed ocean artist Wyland shares his thoughts and meditations, inspired by great nature writers past and present, as a contribution to the conservation of our oceans. This wonderful collection will appeal to art lovers, environmentalists and anyone who has been mesmerized by the sight, sound and smell of the sea.

Code # 7923 • Hardcover • $19.95